The
Green
Vine

The Green Vine

A GUIDE TO WEST COAST SUSTAINABLE, ORGANIC, AND BIODYNAMIC WINE

SHANNON BORG

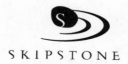

SKIPSTONE

Published by Skipstone, an imprint of Mountaineers Books
Printed in the United States of America
16 15 14 13   1 2 3 4 5

Design and illustrations: Emily Ford
Cover photograph: Chalkboard image courtesy iStockphoto.com
Author photograph: Steve Forman

Library of Congress Cataloging-in-Publication Data
Borg, Shannon.
A guide to West Coast sustainable, organic, and biodynamic wineries / Shannon
Borg.
pages cm
Includes index.
ISBN 978-1-59485-732-4 (ppb)
1. Wineries—Pacific Coast (U.S.)—Guidebooks. 2. Organic wines—Pacific Coast
(U.S.) 3. Organic viticulture—Pacific Coast (U.S.) 4. Sustainable agriculture—Pa-
cific Coast (U.S.) I. Title.
 TP557.B665 2013
641.2'200979—dc23
2013015125

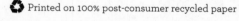 Printed on 100% post-consumer recycled paper

ISBN (paperback): 978-1-59485-732-4
ISBN (ebook): 978-1-59485-733-1

Skipstone books may be purchased for corporate, educational, or other promotional sales. For special discounts and information, contact our sales department
at 800-553-4453 or mbooks@mountaineersbooks.org.

Skipstone
1001 SW Klickitat Way
Suite 201
Seattle, Washington 98134
206.223.6303
www.skipstonebooks.org
www.mountaineersbooks.org

LIVE LIFE. MAKE RIPPLES.

Contents

MAPS 6

   Pacific Northwest Wine Growing Areas 6

   Northern California Wine Growing Areas..................................... 8

   California North Coast Wine Growing Areas (detail) 9

   California Central Coast Wine Growing Areas (detail) 10

Foreword by Randall Grahm 11

Acknowledgments 13

Introduction 15

SUSTAINABILITY AND TERROIR:
THE VIEW FROM 30,000 FEET 17

SUSTAINABILITY IN THE VINEYARD............................. 26

SUSTAINABILITY IN THE WINERY 40

CERTIFICATIONS... 52

A STATE-BY-STATE GUIDE TO GREEN WINEMAKING 83

   How to Use This Guide 86

   Northern California Wineries 90

   Oregon Wineries 116

   Washington Wineries... 152

   Idaho Wineries 186

   British Columbia Wineries................................... 190

Green Vine Resources 196

Index 203

Pacific Northwest Wine Growing Areas

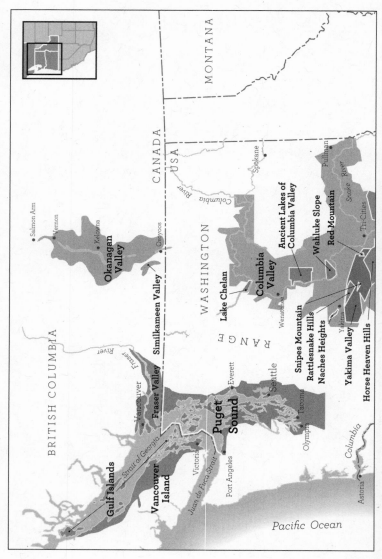

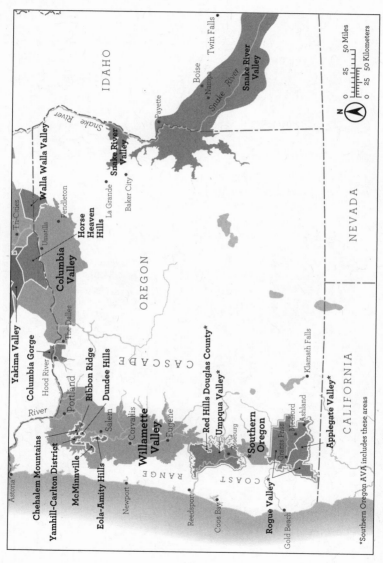

*Southern Oregon AVA includes these areas

Northern California Wine Growing Areas

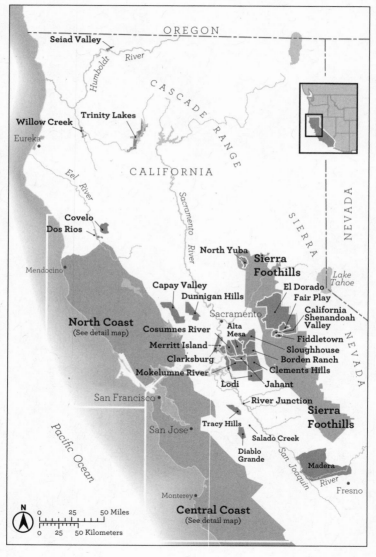

California North Coast Wine Growing Areas (detail)

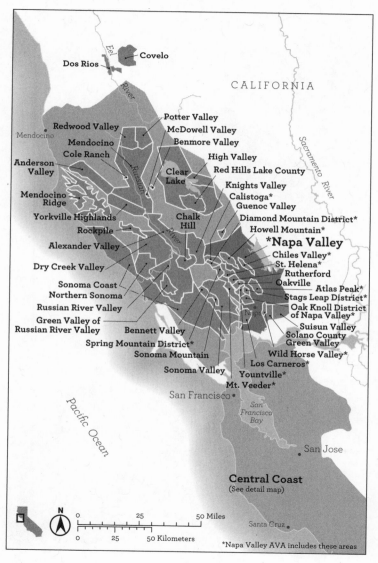

California Central Coast Wine Growing Areas (detail)

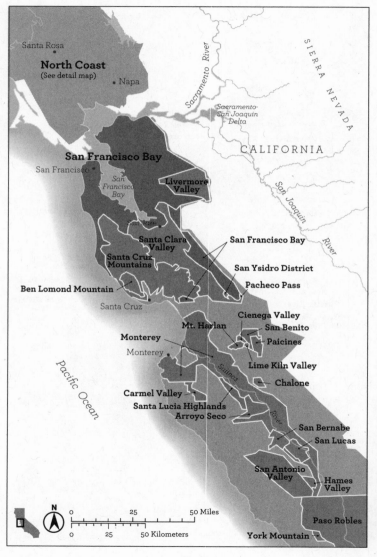

North Coast
(See detail map)

Santa Rosa

Napa

Sacramento River

Sacramento-San Joaquin Delta

SIERRA NEVADA

CALIFORNIA

San Joaquin River

San Francisco Bay

San Francisco

San Francisco Bay

Livermore Valley

San Jose

Santa Clara Valley

San Francisco Bay

Santa Cruz Mountains

San Ysidro District

Pacheco Pass

Ben Lomond Mountain

Santa Cruz

Cienega Valley

San Benito

Mt. Harlan

Paicines

Monterey

Monterey

Lime Kiln Valley

Salinas

Chalone

Carmel Valley

Santa Lucia Highlands
Arroyo Seco

Salinas River

Pacific Ocean

San Bernabe

San Lucas

San Antonio Valley

Hames Valley

Paso Robles

York Mountain

N

0   25   50 Miles

0   25   50 Kilometers

Foreword

A very curious relationship has lately evolved between the mapping of the world of wine and the mapping of the world itself. The latter, with the help of satellite imaging and hyper-connectivity, has grown remarkably detailed and well understood, whereas the former has grown seemingly more obscure and mysterious—new appellations in traditional grape growing regions, new grape growing regions, new/old grape varieties, and radically new/old wine styles. Orange wines! Amphorae? Concrete eggs? (What is one to make of all of this?) The world of wine has grown as dense as *sous-bois*, as beclouded as unfiltered sake. This way be *dunkenfelders*.

For a novice or even relatively experienced wine drinker, how is one to begin to process all of this new information, to create a mental map of the criteria one imagines will bring forth wines that will delight? How do you know what style, aesthetic, or value system of a given wine producer is most resonant with your own sensibility? There is something like a dichotomy (it's actually a false one) that has emerged in the world of wine and it can be parsed several different ways: artisanal versus industrial, laissez-faire versus interventionist, "natural" versus commercial.[1] These dichotomies are perhaps really more like continuums. An utterly controlled or manipulated wine will

. . . .

[1] I am myself taken with the distinction the French make between *vins d'effort* and *vins de terroir*—interventionist wines that bear the strong stylistic imprint of the winemaker as compared to "wines of place," those that seek to capture the ineffable qualities of the site from which the wine derives.

likely be free of commercial flaw, but at the same time may also come off as being somewhat banal, lacking in originality, and perhaps in that elusive quality of "life-force."[2] An entirely "natural" wine, such as an offering from someone like Frank Cornelissen who farms grapes on Mount Etna, is like an exciting, wild ride down a steep road without brakes—certainly not for everyone. For most people, the wine's style, aesthetic, or value system on which it is predicated, is most cordial somewhere between these two polarities. But how is one to even begin to gain a foothold in the mastery of this vast amount of information, opinion, representation/signification of cultural identity that is subsumed in the world of wine?

If you follow the path of becoming a wine geek, you will, almost by definition, at some point be looking for more meaning in your wine. (Not necessarily for wines with higher point scores!) You will likely find a thread that engages you (even if you can't articulate it), and may want to go deep or at least, deeper. Tasting or drinking wine is the precursor to conversation—both with one's fellow imbibers and with the wine itself. The text of this book, along with visits to the vineyards, either in one's imagination or far better, in real time, may well serve as the pretext for many conversations.

—Randall Grahm

. . . .

[2]Life-force or "minerality" (itself, a most elusive term) to my mind, correlates with a wine's ability to tolerate oxidative challenge and speaks to its ability to age gracefully. Wines with these qualities are certainly far more likely to be found from grapes that are grown organically or biodynamically. While no one has yet posited an entirely evident model for the phenomenon of "minerality," there is no question that this phenomenon is linked to grapes grown in soils that are microbiologically robust.

Acknowledgments

For the past dozen years or so, I have had the great good fortune to be able to learn about wine from the most generous winemakers, viticulturists, business owners, wine lovers, editors, and writers in the Washington State wine world. The word "industry" applies to that world in both the sense of a vital, growing branch of our economy and the sense of focused work by dedicated people toward the common goal of making great wine. Writing this book also gave me the chance to visit dedicated winemakers, winegrowers, and wine lovers from Oregon, California, Idaho, and British Columbia. Thanks to all of you for your insight and inspiration.

My great appreciation goes to my editors: Kate Rogers, who first supported this idea, and Janet Kimball, who patiently shepherdessed me through the process. Barry Foy is not only a gifted musician but a gifted copyeditor as well. My editor at *Seattle* magazine, Rachel Hart, has been encouraging and patient beyond belief. Thanks to Kristen Russell and Lisa Wogan as well for their insightful editing.

My gratitude goes out to the many mentors and friends who have continually taught me in so many ways, through their joy for living, their delicious wines, and their insightful advice: Dick Boushey, Rick Small, Virginie Bourgue, Brian Carter, Paul Gregutt, Chris Sparkman, Paul Vandenberg, Shayn Bjornholm, Brennan Leighton, Angie Jabine, Don Townshend, Cole Danehower, Braiden Rex-Johnson, Jen Doak, Jonathan Sindelman, Gabriel Lukeris, Sarah Budge, Guy Harris, Adonis McNiel, Tricia and David Gelles, and all the great people at the Washington Wine Commission.

On a personal note, I am so lucky to have such encouraging friends with amazing palates and a passion for wine, food, and life: Danielle Custer, Monique Barbeau, Linda Stratton, Rose Ann Finkel, Dan Randolph, Dave Mecklenberg, Garland Withers, and Darlin Gray. And thank you, Charles Finkel, for just being yourself. Randall Grahm very generously provided charm and insight—and the foreword for this book.

My friends on Orcas Island have helped me immensely by creating a wonderful community. Much gratitude to my Sirens: Jennifer Brennock, Suzanne Heyd, Jill McCabe Johnson, Cat McCluskey, and Kim Secunda. The ladies at Enzo's sustained me with americanos for innumerable hours: Claire, Jen, Jess, Lily, and of course, Heinz.

And my gratitude goes to Myles Paige, for being so supportive during the writing of this book.

Introduction

I wrote this book because I was confused.

As a wine lover, I wanted to drink delicious wine. As a human being concerned about the complex and disturbing state of affairs on our planet, I wanted to pay more attention to what and how I consumed. Fellow food and wine lovers were starting to ask *Where does my wine come from?* as well as *Where does my food come from?*, and I started hearing about and tasting European biodynamic and organic wines that were delicious and amazing, as opposed to the sketchy possibilities historically found in the "organic wine ghetto" in some wine shops. In addition, I started to see little labels on the backs of wine bottles, presumably indicating that the wines were produced without pesticides or herbicides, or somehow otherwise certified "sustainable."

But I wondered, *What does all this mean?* What is "sustainability" when it comes to wine? I wanted to know more, but my random research was a bit like a kid trying to dig a hole to China: It was messy, and it went on and on and on. Each webpage led me to another. Each academic study led to a whole library. Each book led to another book. Each visit with a winemaker produced new and sometimes contradictory answers.

Of course, that's the glorious nature of learning. But it didn't make up for the fact that there was no one reference guide that could answer the majority of my questions. Most of the books about sustainably made wine were fabulously written memoirs about experiencing the wonders of biodynamics with a winemaker in the vineyard, or they featured tasting notes on incredible wines I couldn't find or couldn't afford.

Still, I realized there was a good reason such a book didn't exist: because the idea was absurd. There is so much information, there are so many organizations, so many vineyards and wineries using varying degrees of organic or sustainable practices, that writing a comprehensive guide to a subject that is growing and changing so rapidly would be impossible. The idea of writing it myself would be especially absurd, since I am not a winemaker, not a viticulturist, not a master sommelier. I am merely a writer who loves wine and has had the chance to meet many great people in the Washington wine industry and write about their excellent products. So, rather than pretending to be the ultimate, comprehensive guide to sustainability as it pertains to wine, this book reflects my personal explorations of the subject of "green" winemaking, and the industries, organizations, and people linked to it.

At present, the wineries of Northern California, Idaho, Oregon, Washington, and British Columbia total more than 4,700, not to mention the thousands of vineyards that supply them with fruit. Many of these producers are beginning to make more sustainable choices, such as lighter packaging, more limited use of herbicides in the vineyard, less irrigation, or avoidance of additives. The selection of wineries in this book is a small, very personal one, highlighting various aspects of the industry, including additives and processes used in winemaking; organics, biodynamics, and biodiversity in the vineyard; species and habitat conservation; water and energy issues; packaging, shipping, and recycling; and by-products of wine production.

I hope you will discover useful resources in these pages that act as starting points for further study, and that you will read, ponder, and respond, so we can continue improving our understanding of this vast and fascinating subject.

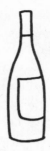

Sustainability and Terroir: The View from 30,000 Feet

Terroir is somewhereness.
—Matt Kramer, wine writer

There is no there there.
—Gertrude Stein

Flying over the Cascade Range from Seattle to Walla Walla is a lesson in winemaking, *terroir* on a large scale, laid out below. We take off from the deep green of conifer forests, up through a dense layer of clouds, breaking into a robin's-egg-blue sky with the snowcapped peaks of Mount Rainier, the blown-out and still growing cinder cone of Mount St. Helens, and sisters Mount Adams and Mount Hood lined up to the south. As we venture eastward, stark contrasts in topography and climate mark our path. Down into the Columbia River Valley, the steep, bare hills and brown scablands have an unfinished look, as if the Great General Contractor in the Sky had run out of money in the middle of a remodeling project. Brown cliffs along the river are sparsely spotted with silver-gray sagebrush, cheatgrass, and wild yellow balsamroot.

The Columbia Valley is a gigantic dry riverbed, and from the plane we see where the water once flowed: rills of darker earth, beautiful soft-brown hills. Then, suddenly, the broad, winding Columbia River cuts, deep blue and glinting, through the landscape below. On one side brown, brown, brown, maybe a little black, a little gold. On the other side, green: Huge fields of agricultural acreage spread out like a patchwork quilt across the Kittitas Valley in pie-shaped patterns in immense round fields of wheat, soybeans, mint, potatoes, and lentils. Pale green and bright yellow stubblefields await new plantings of winter wheat, as well as a new blessing of water from large, wheeled sprinklers that sweep around from a center point to irrigate the crops.

Along the way, the silver glint of hay sheds and silos, the flash of white tarps over piles of baled hay. Stands of poplars are a bulwark against the relentless summer wind, and each town is a gathering of tall trees that look as if they have traveled far to gossip around a giant water cooler. As we descend into Tri-Cities Airport, near the small town of Pasco, we float past fields of endless sagebrush, then the brown rooftops of suburban malls, and parking lots full of cars. We can almost hear, in the distance, the quiet *thup-thup-thup* of the dozens of white wind turbines on the golden-pink hills.

Water formed this waterless landscape. Flying above it, you see its signature in rills where water washed up into the hills as on a gigantic beach, and canyons carved deep into the basalt bedrock laid down millions of years ago when Mount Rainier blew its top.

WATER, WATER, EVERYWHERE

Everything we pass over that is made by human work uses water. "Everything is irrigated," says our tour guide, Jennifer Scott, as she leans forward to peer out the plane window. Scott represents Ste. Michelle Wine Estates (SMWE), a company that includes Chateau Ste. Michelle, Washington's largest winery. She is leading our group to an event sponsored by another SMWE label, Northstar Winery's "Merlot Camp," where we'll learn about all things Merlot from some of the industry's experts, including Northstar winemaker Dave "Merf" Merfield, who produces some rich and elegant wines from vineyards in the Walla Walla Valley.

I'm looking forward to the geeky stuff, like Washington State University (WSU) wine scientist Jim Harbertson's lecture on tannin, color, and taste, and how grapes develop different flavors through their life cycle. I'm looking forward to bending Whitman College geology professor Kevin Pogue's ear about the mysteries of this strange landscape and how it relates to the wine we love. Pogue leads tours of the area, pointing out geological evidence of the floods, such as variegated layers of pale and darker sediment, and connecting the different soil types with the vineyards and wines produced along the route. These range from the mineral-rich (read: nutrient-poor), sun-baked hillsides of Red Mountain, which create bold but complex Cabernet Sauvignon/Merlot blends, to the richer, deeper soils of the relatively wetter, cooler Walla Walla Valley, a source for elegant, earthy Syrahs. And everything in between.

At this point, I know the basics. Formed by a series of immense floods that broke through the ice dams holding back Glacial Lake Missoula, the Columbia Valley was inundated in a mere three days or so by enough water to fill both Lake Erie and Lake Superior. These superflood events happened about every 75 to 100 years, over a period of thousands of years, from about 12,000 to 18,000 years ago. The water carved away the topsoil throughout Eastern Washington, got backed up at Wallula Gap, and left layers of silt along with big

• •

INTERPRETING TERROIR, OR, WINE IS HARD!

Every argument has two sides, right? In the case of winemaking, sustainable or conventional and everything in between, there are as many opinions as there are wines to choose from. From the question of irrigation vs. dry farming, from "greenwashing" to the use of cow horns in biodynamic farming, the discussions are never-ending, and ever-fascinating.

One grower, Hank Beckmeyer of La Clarine Farm in California's Sierra Nevada foothills, pondered questions of the process of winemaking, and terroir in particular, in a blog post called "A Natural Farming Journey at La Clarine Farm," on the farm's website (laclarinefarm.com) and has kindly allowed me to reprint part of it here:

> *Why are the wines made by neighbors sometimes wildly different? If terroir is so site specific, so fixed, why does this happen?*
>
> *It all started to remind me of a quantum field, in that the set of possibilities of a wine (from vineyard to bottle) is (perhaps) infinite. And it strikes me that these possibilities are indeed what we mean by terroir. Terroir (or the terroir-field) is not static and fixed. Rather, it is everything that can be. It relies on an interpretation by someone or something to manifest itself, much like a subatomic particle only has a position when someone is there to observe it. And like a particle, it could be in two different places (or have two different expressions) to two different observers.*
>
> *Each terroir-field embodies this almost limitless set of possible outcomes. Each step in grape growing and in the cellar is a series of decisions that eliminate or restrict certain other possibilities. By choosing A, we may stop B or C from expressing itself. Or choosing A may emphasize other aspects. Our choices, pruning, trellising, vineyard layout, farming, picking, cellar procedures, etc., all serve to define one group of possible outcomes (what we would call its expression of terroir) while restricting others.*

In essence, the farmer/winemaker/vigneron becomes the crucial link in allowing a vineyard, its grapes, and the vintage to express itself. He or she allows a terroir to become explicit.

. . . .

"erratics," huge boulders carried by the glacial ice. Then the water dried up. Over the next centuries, windblown dust known as "loess" blew in from the southern part of Oregon and elsewhere, to deposit a layer of mineral-rich topsoil as fine as talcum powder, from mere inches to many feet thick, across the whole of the Columbia Valley.

Wine lovers in Washington State know about these floods. They talk about how these mineral-rich but organic-poor soils are great for grapevines, making them struggle for water and nutrients. Vines that struggle supposedly produce more intense fruit as they desperately try to send down deep roots and reproduce themselves by generating seed rather than growing shallow roots and more "vigor," or leaf growth, such as a more heavily watered plant would do. Winegrowers are just coming to understand what helps a wine to reflect a particular place, but some, including Bonny Doon Vineyard winemaker Randall Grahm and other winegrowing members of the Deep Roots Coalition (based in Salem, Oregon), think water is the key. "It is essentially a non sequitur to talk about the 'terroir' of an irrigated vineyard, most especially one that is drip-irrigated," Grahm says. "Drip-irrigated vines, unless they are very old, have generally very limited root systems, and as such are not really reflecting the real fingerprint of the site."

So for some, the growing movement toward less water in the vineyard is as much a question of flavor as it is a matter of water conservation. In the Northwest, the Columbia River has been supplying water to human populations since Native people began fishing its waters after the great floods receded about 10,000 years BPT (Before

Present Time), according to the Center for Columbia River History. None of the present day's agriculture—not the wheat, the lentils, the mint, apples, potatoes, wine—nor, for that matter, most of the communities would exist without irrigation, without water. When it comes to vines and wine, a more sustainable—and flavorful—viticulture will be one that seeks to understand the relationship of water to issues surrounding soil and vine health.

LISTENING TO THE LAND

Sustainability is probably the most used, and misused, word of the last decade, and many organizations around the world have struggled to define it. A much referred-to definition appears in *Our Common Future: Report of the World Commission on Environment and Development* (also called the "Brundtland Report," after former Norwegian Prime Minister Gro Harlem Brundtland) published in 1987 by the United Nations World Commission on Environment and Development. It reads, "Sustainable development is development that meets the needs of the present without compromising the ability of future generations to meet their own needs."

In the dry Columbia Valley, generations of Native people sustained themselves through hunting, fishing, and gathering myriad plants, roots, and fruits. Their existence was sustainable, for the most part, until "development" shoved them and their way of life aside. In some of the hottest, driest areas of the United States, Native people grew crops with as little as 10 inches of rain a year, using what we now call "dryland farming" techniques, planting the right crop at the right time of year (according to ancient methods of planting by moon and tide cycles) to ensure water at the right time in the plant's development. They also rotated crops so as to not deplete a field's nutrients and mitigate erosion, a method that is returning, especially in dry areas of California and Washington, where water is at a premium.

The development of this part of the West through the 18th and 19th centuries relied on many things, but the continued supply of water and the health of the soil were paramount, and settlers valued the quality of the land over all other considerations. They dry-farmed too, early on, as the Natives had done for centuries. Some crops, such as winter wheat, can survive on as little as 9 or 10 inches of rain a year, which is why it flourishes in the Russian steppe and the Palouse area of southeastern Washington State.

But these immense fields also suck up the water that falls, which would otherwise feed streams; over the decades there has been a significant reduction in the levels and number of streams in the region. The growth of large-scale agriculture and the introduction of larger farms growing garden crops brought an even greater need for water. The US government began creating systems of irrigation reservoirs, dams, and canals that fed off tributary rivers. An example is the Bureau of Reclamation's Yakima Project (now called the Roza Irrigation District), first surveyed beginning in 1912 and built in the 1930s, which brings water from the Columbia River to 72,000 acres of farms throughout the Yakima Valley that otherwise could barely exist. More than in the lush green Willamette Valley to the south in Oregon, farmers in the Columbia Valley (which includes Idaho's Snake River Valley and part of British Columbia's Okanagan Valley) have worked to control almost every drop of water their crops get. In every wine growing region, farmers face different challenges—and can take advantage of different opportunities—presented by the land. In most of the Columbia Valley farmers don't have to worry about floods, but they do have to deal with wind and heat. Extreme heat is a problem for grapes because, for one thing, they need cool nights to keep from ripening too quickly. In California, where the vast range of landscapes offers an equally vast range of grape-growing environments, climate change may be affecting the conditions with a number of potentially challenging results, and is part of the reason for an ongoing search for new grape-growing sites.

Indeed, every place has its own blessings and its own challenges. Sustainability has everything to do with place. Terroir has everything to do with site. Like all agriculture, viniculture is a partnership between the land and the farmer. The land brings its terroir—poor or rich soil; wind intensity and direction; slope or aspect of hillsides; irrigation, rain, hail, sleet, and sun; soil health, microbes, insects and other fauna; weeds, mildew, fungus, and other flora—and the farmer brings his culture, desires, workers, and decisions. Each grape grower must work with his own resources and with what the specific land and climate has to offer, and many are now choosing to make the least impact possible, to respond to what might be thought of as the vine's desire.

Looking out this plane's window, I realize that what I see below me is an amazing laboratory for the study of sustainability. In this dry region, farmers have created a whole industry out of scablands and a big river. Everything else—soil amendments, pest and disease control, quality decisions, energy for production and packaging, fuel for transport—is brought or created by those who work and manage the land.

If sustainability means the capability of being maintained indefinitely, of meeting environmental, economic, and social needs into the future, then the dreams and desires of those involved must lay the groundwork for it. We have seen what happens when we desire one thing and the land desires another. The examples are many, in the form of environmental disasters ranging from the Johnstown Flood of 1889 to the dust bowl of the 1930s to China's Great Sparrow Campaign of 1958 to the California gold rush, and on through Amazon deforestation, devastation from coal mining in West Virginia, and the current trend of "fracking" for natural gas deposits. The point is that even in the best-intentioned agricultural cultures, the struggle for sustainability is often a struggle with the land itself, to transform it into something other than itself, to manipulate it to follow our own dreams, to find that pot of gold.

In this case, the dream is great wine. The concept of terroir—the aspects of climate, soil, culture, and environment that give a wine its particular taste—obviously has everything to do with place. Wine writer Matt Kramer defines terroir as "somewhereness," and terroir-driven wines can be produced only when the winegrower's and winemaker's desires are aligned with the desires of the land itself. Winegrowers who see dry farming as the best way to produce wines that reflect a particular site focus on sites that can grow grapes with no irrigation, in order to build soil health, root mass, and beneficial mycorrhizal fungi below the surface that aid in water and mineral uptake from the soil. Otherwise, the argument goes, we end up with shallow rooted, over-irrigated, overly manipulated, generic-tasting wine. As Gertrude Stein once said of her hometown of Oakland, California, "There is no there there." Her roots weren't deep; she couldn't hear or feel or taste its "somewhereness." So she exiled herself to the "thereness" of Paris, where she and her art and community and soul felt at home, and flourished.

When it comes to sustainably produced wines with a sense of place, time will tell, and new research is being conducted constantly. But the best outcome seems to occur when growers, makers, and wine lovers take care not to ask something of the place or situation, or the vine, that it can't give. To me, the most interesting wine happens when human desires align with those of the particular grape, in that particular place. When we listen.

Sustainability in the Vineyard

The issue of sustainability in the vineyard encompasses a whole host of topics—soil type, soil amendments, pest and weed control, irrigation—that are at the heart of any discussion of conventional vs. organic vs. biodynamic farming practices. No one has definitive answers, and some current approaches look back in time to traditional farming practices as much as forward, especially among smaller and higher-end vineyards and wineries. Twenty years ago, a story about planting by moon cycles wouldn't be heard at the same cocktail party as one about the latest nitrogen fertilizer. But now, approaches to growing grapes draw from both longstanding traditions and modern research, from both legend and laboratory.

LET'S TALK ABOUT SOIL

Everywhere you look, walk, or taste in the world of wine, people talk about soil. Wine labels tout the slate, flint, tufa, loess, clay, schist, basalt, Jory, and literally hundreds of specific soil types that give a wine that *je ne sais quoi*.

As infused as tasting rooms and wine labels seem to be with this mysterious concept of "minerality," in the realm of viniculture nothing is set, shall we say, in stone. While it's true that different types of soil hold water, temperature, and nutrients differently—clay holds water, gravel drains quickly, light-colored limestone reflects heat up into the vines—it still isn't definitively known how much this all affects taste. In a 1986 study, French researcher Gérard Seguin reported: "As our knowledge stands at the moment, it is impossible to establish any correlation between the quality of wine and the soil content of any nutritive element. . . . If there were such a correlation it would be easy, with the appropriate chemical additives, to produce great wine anywhere."

Since that research, however, there have been many studies on the effects of soil type on the taste of wine. Most interestingly, in 2005 in the journal *Water Science and Technology*, Australian researchers D. E. Mackenzie and A. G. Christy traced the levels of Baumé and Brix (ripeness and sugar levels), pH, total acidity (TA), and phenolic content (a good selection of the things that determine wine flavor) in relation to soil composition in two riesling vineyards. The study "set out to determine whether or not the chemical composition of soil in a vineyard has any influence on the measurable composition of wine grapes produced." They found a whole host of interesting tidbits, including that different types of soils decreased or increased total acidity, pH, and Baumé. For instance, increased clay content "decreases pH and increases TA, possibly reflecting the water-providing properties of clays," and the more calcium and various other minerals available to the plant, the lower the overall Baumé levels.

How does this relate to sustainability? Does it matter if we know whether or not soil composition actually changes taste? The scientists determined that their results "will be useful in developing 'rules' to 'tailor' wine-grape varieties to vineyard sites, and will assist in managing vineyard soils for optimum performance and quality." But in a sense, they also realized that they might be creating a monster. Because of all the talk of minerality expressed in wine, some vineyard managers might be inclined to manipulate the soil by adding "super-phosphate and synthetic chemicals, as well as agricultural lime, dolomite, and gypsum," etc., which may have the short-term effect of improving results but "are known to have long-term harmful effects on the soil." Mackenzie and Christy express hope that future research will show which "naturally occurring additives are best suited to improving the viticultural performance of soils by providing chemical nutrients in a balanced form to which plants are adapted, and doing this in a sustainable way, without risking long-term detriment to the soil and the vineyard."

According to Randall Grahm, naturally deep roots and soil type make all the difference: "The possibility of the expression of terroir ultimately comes down to a very basic ratio: the mass (or more likely the overall surface area) of roots relative to fruit volume. The latter characterization may be more apt as soil types like volcanic, schistous, and calcareous, that have a lot of interior surface area, support much larger mycorrhizal populations. The health and overall mass of the mycorrhizal population are undoubtedly a key element in the articulation of terroir."

GOD MADE DIRT, BUT FARMING MADE IT HURT: THE CONVENTIONAL APPROACH

Different winegrowing philosophies espouse different ways of "managing" the soil. "Conventional" farming is industrialized, usually large-scale farming that developed out of the Industrial Revolution. It focuses on the isolating of nitrogen, phosphorus, and potassium,

(NPK) as elements needed by plants, and synthesizing them for use as "inputs," or chemical fertilizers, making large-scale agricultural production possible. According to Matthew Scully in his book *Dominion: The Power of Man, the Suffering of Animals, and the Call to Mercy*, worldwide food production doubled four times between 1820 and 1975 as a result. In conventional farming, the idea is that soil needs balanced levels of calcium, nitrogen, phosphorus, potassium, and sulfur, and growing crops either adds to or depletes these levels. Therefore, these elements should be replaced in the soil in the form of artificial fertilizers in order to maintain balance. This mode of thinking also sees weeds, insects, rodents, and disease as "problems" solvable by the use of chemicals. But it comes with its own problems: It requires huge amounts of water and energy, for one thing. It can also introduce pests, which are then targeted with hazardous amounts of herbicides and pesticides that can find their way into streams and lakes, polluting the water. And this method depletes topsoil, making it vulnerable to being blown or washed away along with the previously added nutrients.

Following the development of chemicals for use in World War I, an entire agricultural chemical industry grew. The 1909 Haber process was a breakthrough, making use of the reaction of nitrogen gas and hydrogen gas to produce ammonia on an industrial scale. First used in the production of military explosives, it has been employed to produce chemical fertilizers ever since. In the early 20th century, controlling the environment was the popular mindset, and many names of chemical fertilizers or herbicides—Roundup (developed in 1974), Harness, Bullet, Lariat—still speak to an old-school cowboy attitude of farming that is based on the desire for control.

These fertilizers essentially made large-scale farming possible, and their widespread use, according to some, has resulted in the ability to feed the world's growing population. But there is a tremendous downside: The use of chemical fertilizers, pesticides, and herbicides has been a major factor in environmental damage and depletion of natural soil health across the globe. A 2004 US Department of Agriculture (USDA) study of 43 garden crops from 1950 to 1999 suggested that soil depletion in the United States had led to a loss in the nutritional value of our basic foods over the previous 50 years. Amounts of vitamin A, for example, had decreased by 40 to 100 percent in apples, bananas, broccoli, onions, potatoes, and tomatoes.

FINDING A NEW PATH: ORGANIC AND BIODYNAMIC FARMING

When many growers of other crops began transitioning to wine grapes in the 1960s and 1970s, realizing they could make more money, conventional farming was the norm, seen as the key to maximizing production and reducing crop loss. But slowly the industry became aware of environmental issues in the vineyard and the surrounding ecosystems. In Northern California, Frey Vineyards became the first certified-organic vineyard when it joined the California Certified Organic Farmers (CCOF) in 1980 followed by many others throughout the '80s and '90s. In Washington, Bill Powers, the 85-year-old patriarch of Powers Winery, was ahead of his time when he started farming organic grapes in 1982. He had started off using chemical fertilizers, herbicides, and pesticides in the vineyard, but then he realized his kids were running around among the vines. He didn't want them breathing the dust from the chemicals or carrying it into the house on their skin and clothes. So he consulted with WSU viticulturist Walter Clore, who helped him navigate the road to chemical-free, productive grape growing. Powers became the first certified-organic vineyard in Washington State in 1990. Recently honored by the Washington Wine Commission for being an organic pioneer, Powers says his vines keep getting better.

Powers was an outlier, and it will take decades for the organic movement to take hold in grape growing on a large scale in Washington. For the most part, small vineyards have been the first to make small changes. Justin Wylie of Va Piano Vineyards in Walla Walla says of his early days of growing grapes on his 20-acre estate vineyard, "I used to spray everything I had. Now it is completely the opposite." Wylie began working with Rick Trumbull, a soil consultant with a background in the conventional amendments industry who now espouses compost tea over most chemicals. Wylie closely follows the guidelines set out by Vinea: The Winegrowers' Sustainable Trust, a holistic approach that "employs environmentally friendly and socially responsible viticulture practices that respect the land, conserve natural resources," and support biodiversity, among other goals. "I have fewer weeds than ever," he says. "The vineyard is just healthier." Wylie's goal is to build a "premium vineyard" that will last for generations, and he feels that the Vinea approach of promoting responsible relationships with environment, workers, and the community is the best way to set the vineyard and winery up for sustainability and success.

In organic farming, amendments such as farm animal manure, bone meal, blood meal, compost, and earthworm castings all are allowed. They contain high amounts of nitrogen, an important element for plant growth, but in balanced ratios with other elements so as not to create runoff of extra nitrogen. Certain organic chemical amendments, such as biosolids (treated residuals from wastewater treatment), are also used but are controversial. According to the Environmental Protection Agency (EPA), the use of biosolids "is regulated under the Clean Water Act, and is currently subject to concentration limits for the metals arsenic, cadmium, copper, lead, mercury, molybdenum, nickel, selenium, and zinc."

The basic organic tenets show a commitment not only to keeping toxic chemicals out of the vineyard, but to improving the ecosystem through biodiversity and conservation. The USDA National Organic Program (NOP) has set out guidelines for what organic grape growing should look like, and consumers are seeking out these wines through wineries and wine clubs such as the EcoVine Wine Club, which lists these guidelines, based on NOP standards:

- Organic farming helps protect our air, soil, water, and food supply from toxic chemicals and other pollutants.
- Organic grapes are grown without synthetic pesticides, herbicides, fumigants, or fertilizers.
- Organic grapes are never genetically engineered or modified, and [are] never irradiated.
- Organic farming conserves natural resources by recycling natural materials.
- Organic farming encourages an abundance of species living in balanced, harmonious ecosystems.

For many grape growers, organic doesn't go far enough. Biodynamics is a method of farming that has been attracting winegrowers, in France especially, for more than a decade and has been popular in the farming of other crops for much longer than that. Originally a response to a group of Austrian blueberry farmers who wanted to farm without chemicals, biodynamics began as a set of lectures given in 1924 by Austrian philosopher-scientist Rudolph Steiner (who also established the Waldorf education system). In Steiner's view, a biodynamic farm "encourages a view of nature as an interconnected whole, a totality, an organism endowed with archetypal rhythm," according to Demeter International, a certifying organization with a worldwide network of member-inspectors. Paul Beveridge of Wilridge Winery in the Naches Heights AVA (American Viticultural Area) of Washington, says organics is more about what "not to put into the vineyard, while biodynamics is about what should be added to the vineyard to build soil health."

In biodynamics, vines are planted, pruned, and harvested by sun and moon cycles, as in the *Old Farmer's Almanac*, and special preparations containing plants such as nettle, yarrow, chamomile, horsetail, and dandelion, as well as cow manure composted in cow horns, are applied to vineyards to increase healthy microbes and build up the vines' health and immune systems. As for undesirable plant visitors, in place of herbicides, both organic and biodynamic farming enlist the natural systems of the farm to regulate weeds, by planting cover crops among the rows to help increase nitrogen in the soil and keep weeds at bay.

Instead of using poisons to eliminate nasty bugs such as leafhoppers and glassy-winged sharpshooters and critters like gophers, moles, and grape-loving robins, both organic and biodynamic farming encourage natural predators such as swallows, owls, kestrels, and the like. Animals are important to the biodynamic farm, and some farms employ armies of chickens, goats, and sheep to weed-eat to their hearts' content. Farmers are encouraged to plant herbs, grasses, and flowers to attract beneficial insects such as bees, spiders, and ladybugs. And according to Wilridge's Paul Beveridge, it works. He composts and works with green manure (cover crops that are then reworked into the soil); legumes such as cowpeas, soybeans, sweet clover; and nonleguminous crops such as millet, sorghum, and buckwheat. Beveridge also mixes and sprays preparations according to Demeter USA guidelines, following moon and sun cycles. "My vineyard gets more healthy each year as we build the soil," he says. "The biggest difference I find is that the wines are more aromatic than nonbiodynamic wines I've made." By contrast, conventional farming's monoculture landscape is relatively bare of trees, bushes, herbs, and grasses, all of which could serve as habitat for a wide range of beneficial animals and insects.

Many winegrowers, including Bill Powers, admit that choosing the right site is all-important when it comes to sustainability. "We have a big advantage being in a desert, where you don't have to worry about humidity," Powers says. "And the pests that cause the most problems, the leafhoppers and spider mites, well, they aren't a problem, because when you stop using chemicals to kill them, you stop killing the good bugs, too." The natural balance of predator and prey is restored, and overgrowth of harmful insects decreases—not to nil, but to a manageable level.

THE "WOO-WOO" CONTROVERSY

Admittedly, biodynamics is not every vintner's cup of compost tea. Many people see it as a pagan-inspired, ritualistic "voodoo-woo-woo" way of making wine. According to Katherine Cole, wine writer for *The Oregonian* and advocate of biodynamic wine, in her book *Voodoo Winemaking: Oregon's Astonishing Biodynamic Winegrowers*, the contemporary revival of the biodynamic movement began in 1989 when French microbiologist Claude Bourguignon produced studies claiming that the soils of Burgundy had less microbial life than those of the Sahara Desert and proposed biodynamics as an answer. After tasting the magnificent wines that are now coming from biodynamic vineyards in that region, including the iconic Romanée-St-Vivant and Clos de la Roche vineyards, many growers began converting to biodynamics themselves. Organic composting may have been enough to heal the soil, but the fact that the famous Domaine Leflaive vineyard did side-by-side comparisons of organic and biodynamic wines and then converted to the latter has transformed the region into biodynamic believers.

But there is a strong streak of mysticism in the method, and some practitioners become true believers while others choose to ignore the more out-there ideas. Renowned producer of certified-biodynamic wines Nicolas Joly lays out some of the fundamentals of Rudolph Steiner's ideas in *Biodynamic Wine, Demystified* and other books. He speaks of the four forces of energy—warmth (fruit), light (flower), liquid (leaf), and mineral (root)—mediated by solar forces of levity and earthly forces of gravity. Each plant's individual form dictates its dominant energy. For instance, because of its broad leaves, small roots, and thin stalks, the bright-green stinging nettle has heat and light energy as its dominant driving forces; a homeopathic spray made from its leaves brings that energy to the vines, "enlivening" them.

These ideas are traceable to the German scientist/philosopher Johann Wolfgang von Goethe, who looked back to Aristotle's writings and interpreted them through the scientific knowledge of his own time. There's much more to Steiner's fascinating practices and concepts than can be explained here, and the reading is entertaining if nothing else. Might I suggest reading Joly while enjoying a glass of certified-biodynamic Montinore Pinot Gris? (See the "Demeter Certified Biodynamic Preparations" sidebar in the Certifications chapter.)

SALMON, SALMON EVERYWHERE

With the expansion of the Oregon-based Salmon-Safe program, the Washington wine industry is slowly coming up to speed with Oregon and California in sustainable agriculture. Salmon-Safe winegrowing requires that vineyards commit to not polluting ground and surface water that may flow into streams and rivers where salmon live and spawn, thereby helping to preserve salmon habitat. Each vineyard must meet guidelines specific to efficient irrigation and water conservation measures, erosion control, integrated pest management (IPM), and native vegetation and habitat management.

Vineyards across Washington State are gaining their Salmon-Safe certification, including Novelty Hill Winery's estate vineyard, Stillwater Creek, the first Columbia Valley vineyard to acquire the designation. The 245-acre vineyard is one of the steepest sites in the state, with hills running at 22 percent grade in places. This makes for great drainage, but if herbicides and pesticides are used, they can too easily drain off this large vineyard into ground and surface water that eventually ends up in the Columbia River, just a few miles away.

Other, smaller vineyards are even closer to riparian habitats. For instance, àMaurice Cellars and its neighbor Abeja both have vineyards near Mill Creek, a sensitive watershed east of Walla Walla where historically bull trout, steelhead, and Chinook salmon returned to spawn. The last significant Chinook run was in 1925, but many groups have been working on this project in recent years, including the Confederated Tribes of the Umatilla Indian Reservation, who have attempted to restock this stream.

In 2005, Kooskooskie Dam, about 10 miles upstream from àMaurice and Abeja, was removed, and habitat improvements all along the creek into downtown Walla Walla are ongoing. "We want to get the salmon up to the great habitat at Kooskooskie," says Brian Burns, project manager for the dam removal project sponsored by the Tri-State Steelheaders fisheries enhancement group. Stewardship Partners, a Seattle nonprofit that helps private landowners restore and preserve their natural landscapes, has produced a handy pocket-sized

SOME FAVORITE SALMON-SAFE WINES

Buty Conner Lee Vineyard Chardonnay, Columbia Valley
This lush and fragrant Chardonnay explodes with ripe peach and soft spice, and a touch of ginger on the finish for an excellent food wine. Pairs with: Pumpkin soup with nutmeg and crème fraîche.

Novelty Hill Roussanne, Stillwater Creek Vineyard, Columbia Valley
This southern Rhône varietal is usually blended but is a delight on its own. The Stillwater Creek Vineyard enjoys the perfect climate for bringing this warm weather grape to its full potential, showing aromas and flavors of peach and spice, along with a soft mouthfeel that lends a lushness to this dry wine. Pairs with: Roast chicken with preserved lemon.

Abeja Cabernet Sauvignon, Columbia Valley
Lively aromas of boysenberry and black cherry are followed by more lush dark fruit on the palate, integrated vanilla and toast. This 100 percent Cabernet Sauvignon is grown on Abeja's estate vineyard on the banks of Mill Creek just east of Walla Walla. Pairs with: Braised lamb shoulder with shaved fennel and white beans.

Pepper Bridge Cabernet Sauvignon, Walla Walla Valley
This blend, usually made from Cabernet Sauvignon, Merlot, Cabernet Franc, Malbec, and Petit Verdot, comes from two Salmon-Safe vineyards—Seven Hills and Pepper Bridge's Estate Vineyard. An incredibly balanced and elegant wine, showing dark plum, toast, coffee, and black cherry flavors. Pairs with: Roast lamb with red wine reduction sauce.

card listing Salmon-Safe wines, so you can choose one when you are out to dinner at a restaurant or shopping at your local wine shop.

Habitat improvement along a river or stream requires the commitment of everyone along the way. Historically, riverbank neighbors such as wheat farmers, wineries, and orchards used herbicides and pesticides that would end up getting washed into the streams, but that is changing. To date, more than half of the vineyards in the Walla Walla area are certified Salmon-Safe, and the number is growing across the state.

Anna Schafer, winemaker and partner at àMaurice Cellars, says that her family's commitment to sustainable winegrowing was not negotiable. "Before we planted our vineyard, we just 'grew dirt' for two years," she says, describing the process the vineyard went through to repair damage done from wheat and pea rotation on the land—and to gain Vinea and Salmon-Safe certification in 2006. The vineyard's manager, Ken Hart, who manages several vineyards in the area and is a big proponent of sustainable winegrowing practices, worked to improve the soil by adding compost, compost teas, soft rock phosphate, kelp, and other organic matter to bring it back into balance. "We agree that making sure the vineyard doesn't disrupt or pollute our water system is essential to making our industry sustainable, and to making great wine," says Schafer. "We are proud that we are a part of the solution and are creating a sustainable vineyard for the future."

Dry farming is a relatively new trend in grape growing and an old trend in agriculture. Once, farmers—and grape growers—planted their crops and hoped for rain. Now, irrigation taken from streams and rivers brings water, but with climate change and the many environmental problems surrounding water usage, and since grapes don't need much water, some vineyard managers are trying to avoid watering at all, in order to encourage the vines' roots to extend deep into the soil for sustenance and to develop healthy mycorrhizal (fungi) populations, on the vines' roots, which helps facilitate mineral absorption. The Deep Roots Coalition of Oregon is a group that encourages dry-farming techniques, following the lead of French wineries such as Burgundy's renowned Domaine de la Romanée-Conti, which does not irrigate vines after they are established. This method ensures that the vines grow slowly and develop long roots, and is more in tune with the natural cycle of weather, which founder John Paul of Cameron Winery feels is what is missing when vines receive regular water. At the moment, the Deep Roots Coalition has 17 members: Anderson Family Vineyard, Ayres Vineyard, Beaux Frères, Belle Pente Vineyard, Brick House Vineyards, Cameron Winery, Crowley Wines, Evening Land Vineyards, Evesham Wood Winery, Eyrie Vineyards, Illahe Vineyards, J. Christopher Wines, J. K. Carriere Wines, Matello Wines, Patricia Green Cellars, John Thomas Winery, and Westrey Wine Company. These wineries are committed to exploring the benefits of dry farming, with the goal of producing wines as great as the best in Burgundy.

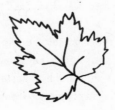

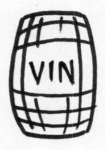

Sustainability in the Winery

Winemakers often say, "Wine is made in the vineyard." But when it comes to getting wine into your glass, it's all about the winery. And if you are concerned about the purity of your food—and wine *is* food—knowing more about how a winery works will help you make more informed choices.

In a nutshell, grapes are brought into the winery at harvest, sorted and pressed, and are left to ferment (and, for reds, to sit on the skins to develop color). This process can take from days to weeks. Once fermentation is over, the wine is "racked" into a barrel, for reds and barrel-raised whites like Chardonnay, or a tank, for many whites. After a certain period of time (up to two years or more for reds or as little as a few days for unoaked whites), the wine is filtered and bottled.

Seems like a simple process, right? But in reality it isn't simple at all. In fact, there is an endless number of choices a winemaker makes, all of which can affect the wine and how sustainable it is. Throughout the winemaking, myriad things can go wrong ("stuck" fermentation, overly high alcohol, low acidity, high tannins, microbial or yeast problems), and the winemaker has to decide how to handle any of these issues, whether conventionally, organically, or biodynamically. In addition to having to solve problems, she also faces decisions about the process of creating the kind of wine she desires. From a light, fresh, unoaked Pinot Gris to a *sur lie*, barrel-fermented Chardonnay to a Beaujolais Nouveau with aromas of bubblegum and strawberry to a deep, rich Bordeaux-style blend aged in French oak barrels for 36 months, the choices are endless. To achieve the desired end requires numerous choices as to the means.

MY CHEMICAL ROMANCE

Much of winemaking is chemistry, and for centuries winemakers have used naturally occurring products to aid in the traditional winemaking process. For instance, albumen, or egg white, can be used (about three to four whites per 25-gallon barrel) to "fine" wine, or help remove cloudiness, as it draws all the little bits of grape skin and pulp to it. Isinglass (a collagen from the dried swim bladders of fishes) or milk protein (casein) can also be added to wine to fine it. Bentonite, an incredibly absorbent weathered volcanic ash clay is also used to absorb excess proteins from wine. Wheat paste is sometimes used to seal oak barrels. These may not be substances, however, that you want to put into your body, depending on your sensitivities or your mindset. People with gluten intolerance or egg allergies, as well as vegans or people with a desire for pure food, may consume wine without knowing that it contains these substances, as there is no law that requires wineries to disclose them on the label.

However, in an article called "The Natural Wine Movement," published on foodtourist.com, Sue Dyson and Roger McShane trace a rise in "manipulated" wines over the past few decades: "Stainless steel started to replace wooden barrels, chemicals became the norm for controlling weeds and disease, additives became the norm rather than the exception, technology such as reverse osmosis machines and roto-fermenters became the tools of winemakers and commercial yeasts started to stamp their indelible flavors on wines."

The "natural wine" movement, as it exists in France as a "beyond organic" philosophy, focuses on keeping wine pure. Certified Organic, Demeter Certified Biodynamic, LIVE (Low Input Viticulture and Enology), and other certifications also eschew chemical fertilizers, herbicides, and pesticides.

From the consumer's perspective, this may seem pretty easy to do—wine is just grape juice and yeast, right? Well, yes and no. Just like inputs (fertilizers) in the vineyard, there are all sorts of additives used in the winery after the grapes have been brought in and fermentation has begun. A whole host of chemicals, both synthetic and natural, are used to start and stop certain processes, to add acidity and tannins or soften them, reduce alcohol, fix flaws, and so on. In her excellent book *Naked Wine: Letting Grapes Do What Comes Naturally*, wine writer Alice Feiring lists at least 80 US-approved additives for wine, for juice, and "for the treatment of distilling material," as used in port and other fortified wines. And as Feiring says, "These are just the 'approved' ones."

Beyond the natural items, which include yeasts, of course, soy flour, and oak particles, other approved, chemically produced additives include potassium metabisulfite, which produces sulfites and helps prevent oxidation and refermentation. Polyvinylpyrrolidone (PvPP) is used in white wine to keep it from turning brown through oxidation and in rosé to lighten the color. Divergan F (another PvPP) keeps whites and rosés from turning cloudy when cold.

WHAT'S IN MY WINE?

The more you know about how natural or manipulated the winemaking process is, the more understanding you'll have of the kinds of flavors to expect from your wine. The main thing is to be as well informed as possible about what you are buying. Here are a few good questions to ask of your winemaker or purveyor:

- Is this wine made with commercial yeast, or is it fermented without any added yeast? Natural yeast is sometimes unpredictable and commercial yeasts are often used to create certain tastes and aromas.
- Has this wine undergone malolactic fermentation? This heating process is applied to almost all reds and some whites (mostly Chardonnay); it softens acids, adding a buttery or creamy texture and flavor.
- What level of sulfites (naturally occurring or commercial) have been added to this wine? Some say that sulfites act like salt—adding a little brings out flavor— as well as keep the wine from spoiling during transit. But too much can make the wine lose its fruit and complexity. If a wine is certified biodynamic, organic, or LIVE, permissible levels of sulfites are strictly laid out.
- Are there any other flavor-changing additives or processes used in this wine? Oak chips, ascorbic acid, tannin enhancers and reducers, as well as processes like reverse osmosis for alcohol reduction, are used to change a wine's flavor.

I'm not saying that these ways in which wine can be manipulated are necessarily good or bad. But they all affect the wine, and you may want to know about it, especially if you want to pair food with wine on the basis of their most natural elements, flavors, and complexity.

Perhaps the quintessential "Frankenwine" tool isn't an additive at all, but a process. The "spinning cone" is a centrifuge that, to put it simply, extracts all flavor compounds from wine, then some of the alcohol. The flavor components are then mixed back in. This process is called "flavor management" and is used mostly when wines are so ripe that the sugars create overly high alcohol levels. The ability to remove some of the alcohol allows winemakers to use the ripest fruit possible, creating big, fruity wines without the high levels of alcohol that would naturally occur.

When the natural wine movement in France and, increasingly, abroad began to take hold, this was part of what winemakers were resisting: not just pesticides, herbicides, and fertilizers in the field, but flavor management and manipulation of wine that compromised not only the integrity of the product but the taste as well. In the 1970s and '80s, French winemaker and research chemist Jules Chauvet led the "vin naturel" movement, which rejected the use of any chemical additives in wine, as well as commercial yeasts. According to French natural winemaker Eric Texier in a discussion on winedisorder.com, Chauvet felt that commercial yeasts distort the expression of terroir. He favored letting the naturally occurring yeasts in the grapes create an "aromatic fermentation" that adds flavor to the wine. Rather than forcing wine to be a certain flavor profile, which may involve overripening grapes to develop rich fruit flavors many people (and critics) love, and then using certain yeasts to add specific flavors followed by spinning the excess alcohol from the wine, the natural winemaker tries to guide the wine to be what it wants to be, hoping that a good growing environment and minimal manipulation—not even adding commercial yeast—will allow the fruit and the land to express their true nature.

If this sounds idealistic, it is. But as with the Slow Food movement—which began in 1986 as journalist Carlo Petrini's reaction to a McDonald's restaurant being built on Rome's Spanish Steps—the natural wine movement in France began as a reaction to overly manipulated wines. Both movements soon took the form of philosophies all their own, with the goals of reviving and protecting tradition, culture, and good taste.

THE POWER OF POSITIVE DRINKING

So far, we've barely gotten out of the tank and barrel. But a winery is much more than that. Most wineries, behind the Italian columns or rustic wood-finished tasting rooms, are industrial buildings meant for work. They have to be heated and cooled, for example, just like any other workplace. If a tank or its environment gets too hot in the summer, strange things can happen to the delicate process of fermentation and aging. Most wineries require a fair amount of energy for climate control, which uses natural resources and costs money.

If special certification programs such as USDA Certified Organic or Demeter Certified Biodynamic are helping wineries improve their vineyard health and eliminate toxic chemicals, certification programs such as LEED (Leadership in Energy and Environmental Design) are addressing issues in the winery of construction, water and energy use, chemical products, and more. Using a 100-point system, LEED rates buildings in the categories Sustainable Sites, Water Efficiency, Energy and Atmosphere, Materials and Resources, and Indoor Environmental Quality, with extra points for Innovation in Design and Regional Priority. Even many wineries that aren't involved in this program are finding ways that work for them to lower their energy use.

Regional organizations such as the Oregon Wine Board and the Oregon Environmental Council are also working to reduce energy use and greenhouse gas emissions. These two organizations have created the Carbon Neutral Challenge, with a goal of making Oregon wineries carbon neutral, through first assessing their energy use and then helping them reduce it, and finally incorporating carbon offsets to reach the goal of carbon neutrality.

Again, for a growing number of winegrowers, nature is smartest. For centuries, wineries and cellars have been built underground, because most cellars maintain a constant temperature of 55°F or so. That saves a lot of energy in warmer climates and helps avoid fluctuating temperatures, which are one of the biggest enemies of wine. Many wineries are learning from history and building underground barrel rooms. For instance, winemaker Keith Pilgrim of Terra Blanca Winery on Washington State's Red Mountain repurposed several huge metal arches from a federal building project and used them in his "cut and cover" cellar, first digging into the side of a hill, then erecting the arches over the space and covering them back up with soil. His capacious barrel room stays cool without air conditioning.

- -

THE TASTE CONTROVERSY

In the early phase of the organic movement, organic wine did not have a reputation for outstanding quality or flavor. Many wineries left the words "organically grown grapes" off the label so as not to be relegated to the organic section of the wine shop. Now, though, many winemakers are transitioning to organics and biodynamics precisely because of taste. In 2004, *Fortune* magazine reported on a group of 10 top sommeliers and wine critics who compared 10 pairs of wines in similar price ranges and from vineyards in the same areas. Of each pair, one wine was conventionally farmed and the other biodynamic. Of the 10 pairs, 9 of the winners were biodynamic wines, notable for the purity of their aromatics and the freshness of their flavors.

But it has become clear that just because a wine can be labeled "organically grown" doesn't mean sustainable practices carry over to the winery. There can still be a lot of manipulation with additives and processes that change the nature of this "natural" wine. That is why there are so many different levels and types of organic and other certifications (we'll go into the specifics later). The main thing for consumers is to keep asking questions of wine shop owners, winemakers, and winegrowers. The consumer must keep the conversation going.

. . . .

In 2002, Sokol Blosser winery, in Willamette Valley, Oregon, was the first Silver LEED–certified, underground, naturally cooled barrel cellar in the United States, when there were only 37 other LEED buildings in the country. In 2005, Stoller Vineyard gained the Gold LEED certification for its solar-supported, multilevel, gravity-flow winery built into a hillside. Gold LEED–certified Hall Winery in Napa Valley has more than 35,000 square feet of solar panels on top of its barrel rooms. If all this sounds time-consuming and incredibly expensive, it is, but that hasn't kept many wineries from installing solar panels, as well as creating gravity-flow systems to move the wine through the process, rather than pumping it.

Many wineries are going solar, especially in California (and more and more in Eastern Washington). The solar panels aren't cheap, but even for a small winery, they often pay for themselves in the form of lower power bills within 10 years of their installation. Many small wineries have a few solar panels to power equipment and run air conditioning or heating units, but a lot of larger ones are going solar big-time. One such megawinery is Constellation Brands, which owns Black Box, Ravenswood, Robert Mondavi Private Selections, and many more brands around the world. Constellation has installed 17,000 solar panels in four wineries in California, for an energy savings equivalent to 9 million miles not driven annually or 225 million miles not driven during the next 25 years. This saves tons of money over the years, of course, resulting in what you might call a wine-win situation.

Each grape is really a little solar power plant in itself, and traditionally, grape growers have "powered" their compost piles with pomace (skin, seeds, stems, and pulp left over from wine production), as well as using it to produce grappa, brandy, eau de vie, and other distilled liquors. Several companies in California, Oregon, and Washington are also using the seeds to produce delicious grapeseed oils. Beyond these uses, the millions of tons of grape pomace from wine production may also be finding a place in the world of biofuel: In Canada, Constellation Brands' Jackson-Triggs and Inniskillin wineries have partnered locally with Vandermeer Greenhouses to use leftover grape skins for energy production to power homes and businesses in the Niagara region of eastern Canada. And a company in New York, Seneca BioEnergy, is beginning to process pomace into grapeseed oil, biodiesel, and soil amendments.

A PACKAGE DEAL

Once the wine is made, it has to get to our glass. Again, choices ensue—from bag to bottle to box. The norm for the past 150 years has been the bottle, in sizes from the diminutive piccolo, or split (187 milliliters, about a twentieth of a gallon), to the grand Melchizedek (30 liters, nearly 8 gallons) and two dozen sizes in between, with the 750 milliliter "standard" (about a fifth of a gallon) as the norm. Before that, the container of choice might have been a barrel in a café, a leather bag, or an amphora, but time marches on, and now we have a billion-bottle-a-year disposal problem, not to mention all the cardboard boxes that make those bottles easy to ship. A glass wine bottle weighs about a pound, 40 percent of the gross weight of a bottle of wine. So lower-weight bottles can make a big difference: Adelsheim Vineyards in Oregon, for instance, uses bottles that weigh 3 ounces less than bottles it used in the past. That adds up, and each truckload of wine now

PUT A CORK IN IT

Cork is one of the most sustainable materials around, since cork trees can live for up to 300 years and the bark is harvested every 9 to 12 years. There are more than 6.6 million acres of Mediterranean cork forest across Portugal, Spain, Algeria, Morocco, Italy, Tunisia, and France, with a level of biodiversity second only to that of the Amazonian rainforest. As an argument against screwcaps, the cork industry has noted, "In comparison to a natural cork, 24 times more greenhouse gases are released and over 10 times more energy is used when making one screw cap." But there are 13 billion natural corks produced each year, and the industry is threatened by the use of other closures. If the cork industry dies, those forests are in danger of being eradicated, as well as the plants and endangered species, such as Iberian lynx, Iberian imperial eagle, and Barbary deer, that live in them. Thousands of workers are supported by the cork harvesting industry as well—many families have worked harvesting cork for generations.

Cork forests are drawing the attention of several different organizations that work to encourage sustainable harvesting practices. One company, ReCORK by Amorim (www.recork.org), gathers used corks through wineries to keep the carbon footprint low on shipping and recycles them into beautiful shoes made by the footwear company SOLE.

Another organization, Cork ReHarvest, is a 501(c)(3) nonprofit that collects and recycles corks, as well as creating the "Real Cork Inside" assurance program, which displays a little cork acorn and the words "Real Cork Inside" on bottles, so people can tell that the closure is cork and not plastic before buying. In response to the problem of "corked" bottles of wine, or corks tainted with 2,4,6-trichloroanisole (TCA), Cork ReHarvest says that although the industry initially responded slowly, now there is a much lower chance of getting a tainted cork; it claims 1 percent of corks are tainted. Corks, unlike plastic stoppers or screwcaps, are renewable and recyclable, and the cork industry supports thousands of jobs in harvesting, production, and recycling. You can find additional information from the Cork Forest Conservation Alliance (www.corkforest.org).

weighs 2,600 pounds less than in previous years, meaning more wine can fit on one truck and less fuel is used in the shipping process.

Trying to find out how many glass bottles we use each year is like trying to find, well, a wine bottle in a Portlandia landfill. In 2011, in the United States we drank 291 million cases of wine. That translates to 3.5 billion bottles, give or take. We recycle millions of tons of bottles each year. But the sad truth is, unless you live in a community where aggressive recycling is the norm, many millions of tons of glass bottles are made, shipped empty, filled with wine, shipped again using fuel and creating greenhouse gases, stored on shelves in controlled-climate shops, purchased, driven home, drunk, and discarded into a landfill. According to a 2009 EPA report, only 18.1 percent of wine and liquor bottles are recovered (of 1.7 million tons generated). Beer drinkers do better than that: Beer bottles are recycled at a 39 percent rate out of 6 million tons generated. That, frankly, is still pretty bad. But we can do better, wine drinkers!

Many people are working on this problem. Glass recycling actually has gone down in the past decade, partially because we are drinking more wine from containers other than glass. Bag-in-a-box, lighter Eco-Glass bottles, refillable containers, jugs, wine kegs, plastic PET bottles (recyclable, made from polyethylene terephthalate), and other types of packaging have become much more accepted, even in the past decade. The fastest-growing new packaging is actually one of the oldest: Tetra Pak is a Swedish company that started making its "aseptic" milk cartons in the 1950s to help milk stay fresh. The most famous wines to be put into Tetra Prisma aseptic cartons on a large scale are probably Boisset's French Rabbit and Constellation's Vendange, in 2005. Using a Tetra Prisma carton, which weighs 40 grams, means 92 percent less packaging for the same wine, 80 percent less greenhouse gas, 40 to 50 percent lower transportation cost, and 54 percent less energy consumption than that of a glass bottle throughout the entire life cycle.

So why don't we drink all of our wine out of a Tetra Pak? Say it with me: Romance! Most winemakers—and wine drinkers—would say that drinking wine from an airtight box is about as romantic as drinking wine from a football helmet. But a planet full of garbage isn't that romantic either. In a few hundred years, ideas about romance and beauty will probably shift anyway. And when it comes down to it, the romance actually comes from swirling the wine in your glass and experiencing its aromas and flavors, in good company.

One company has embraced the "romance of the Tetra Pak" with vigor. Yellow+Blue (get it, Green?) is the brainchild of former Kermit Lynch wine representative Matthew Cain, who struck out on his own to fill a niche he felt was being ignored by the industry. He imports great organic wines and sells them in his Y+B Tetra Pak boxes. His website points out, "When it comes down to it, there is no difference between packaging wine in a Tetra Pak and putting wine in a bottle. It's true. No magic potion or formula that makes bottled wine better. No secret rituals in the vineyard or winery. No difference at all."

People talk about aging wines with the traditional bottle-and-cork method as being better. It would be interesting to use various kinds of packaging and closures—bag-in-a-box, Vino-Lok glass cork, Stelvin closure (screwcap), Tetra Prisma Aseptic pouch, aluminum can, and traditional—to store the same wine, and see which of them make for better aging and longer life. A 25-year-old Y+B? Bring it on!

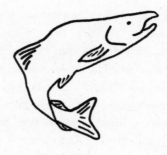

Certifications

The best fertilizer is the farmer's footsteps.
—*The Old Farmer's Almanac*

All of the certifications in the world won't guarantee great, or even good, wine. But when farmers are out in their vineyards working toward and showing long-term commitment to sustainable practices, it is definitely an indication to the consumer that they are dedicated to keeping their vineyards as natural as possible, which translates into purer wine.

But controversy surrounds every aspect of organic, biodynamic, and even sulfite-free wine and what they all mean to the environment, the winemaker, and the consumer. A controversial 2011 study reported in the *Annals of Internal Medicine* on organic vs. nonorganic food stated that there is no marked nutritional benefit to organics. It isn't too surprising that a reader of this report might wonder, Why organic? After all, if the nutrition isn't better, and the taste may or may not be that much better, and yet the price is higher, why bother?

The fact is, for people who choose organic wine, food, and other products, nutrition is only part of the issue. Claiming there's no difference in nutrition might make for an influential, if unfortunate, sound bite, but it misses the more important question: Why should we care about how our food is produced? The answer is that so many related issues, such as energy use in production, biodiversity, monoculture, packaging waste, habitat conservation, water purity, air quality, and fuels used in shipping represent challenges that are becoming increasingly essential to face, both on a local and a global scale.

In a 2009 article in the *New York Times*, two years before the 2011 kerfuffle, Mark Bittman argued that eating organic, which, he says, "seems to have become the magic cure-all, synonymous with eating well, healthfully, sanely, even ethically," actually offers "no guarantee of any of that. And the truth is," he continues, "that most Americans eat so badly—we get 7 percent of our calories from soft drinks, more than we do from vegetables; the top food group by caloric intake is 'sweets'; and one-third of the nation's adults are now obese—that the organic question is a secondary one." He says, "It's not unimportant, but it's not the primary issue in the way Americans eat." Slow Food encourages people to buy "Local First, Organic Next"—to support local farmers and help make a closer connection between our food and the places we live, rather than purchasing an organic tomato in January that was grown in Chile and shipped to Seattle.

Is the question of organics or any other "sustainable" labeling only a secondary question for wine as well? Wine, like food, is about choices. Just like farmers of our food, winegrowers and winemakers make a thousand choices about the planting, growing, harvesting, processing (fermentation, aging), and bottling, storing, marketing, selling, and shipping of their grapes and wine—all very deliberate decisions, and all of which may help create a mediocre wine or a great bottle. And we make choices in the wines we buy. Many wine drinkers I know buy a range of wines depending on the occasion, from cheap, kangaroo-emblazoned, commercially produced Australian Chardonnay for a company barbecue to expensive, local, biodynamically grown, super-premium Syrah for a special birthday.

Our choices are driven sometimes by price, sometimes by our values, and always by the complexities of contemporary society. In European wine, the organic and especially the biodynamic movements have been going strong for over a decade. Although only about 2 percent of European vineyards are organic, compared with 4.7 percent of the total European agricultural picture, the trend toward natural and sustainable wine is growing. And why? Follow the money, of course. In 2008, US sales of organic food products rose to $24.6 billion, and the market has grown an average of 20.2 percent per year. The growing number of winegrowers and winemakers who are eliminating chemical herbicides, pesticides, and fertilizers and lowering energy usage are making those choices for more than just taste. Just like wine drinkers, winegrowers and winemakers are being driven toward more pure wine by a multitude of forces, from finances to philosophy to family.

WHO IS THAT MAN BEHIND THE CURTAIN?

With all these choices, how does the conscientious consumer, standing in the grocery store aisle at 5:45 PM, judge which bottle to choose? Certification labels, awarded by administrative organizations that inspect vineyards and wineries for compliance with various requirements, are a starting point. However, they are not without problems of their own.

Certifications abound, but it's hard to know exactly how meaningful they are. The sheer number of them on winery websites and the backs of bottles these days is daunting: USDA Certified Organic, Salmon-Safe, Demeter Certified Biodynamic (a registered trademark), Napa Green, LIVE Certified, Oregon Certified Sustainable, Fish Friendly Farming, Bee Friendly Farming, to name a few. And the details of these programs are often fuzzy, if not completely mysterious, to the average consumer. When it comes to sustainable and organic farming standards worldwide, there is not just one set of them, not just one organization deciding this or that. The list of organizations involved is a crazy alphabet soup of intimidating bureaucracy. Standards are often set by governmental agencies—the USDA, for instance—with certification done by regional inspecting organizations such as Oregon Tilth. This is why, on wine labels, and many food labels as well, we see all sorts of logos, all with the intention of making things clearer for the consumer. But things are often as clear as, well, compost.

There is a movement to standardize organics across the globe. Internationally, a few organizations, such as the International Organization for Biological and Integrated Control of Noxious Animals and Plants (IOBC), support research that is then utilized by certifying bodies around the world to set standards. A coalition of organizations—the Food and Agriculture Organization of the United Nations (FAO), the International Federation of Organic Agriculture Movements (IFOAM), and the United Nations Conference on Trade and Development (UNCTAD)—has formed GOMA, or Global Organic Market Access, which works toward creating harmony across all certifying agencies from country to country with the IFOAM Family of Standards and will work with COROS, the Common Objectives and Requirements of Organic Standards, and a few other organizations to standardize organic requirements.

See what I mean? How can a chemical-free carrot be so complicated?

All this organization, and all these acronyms, may or may not be a good thing. Yes, creation of an easier, more understandable system of what is required for farms to be compliant, especially across international borders, is great. But many farmers and winegrowers say these large organizations often don't understand the variability and different needs of small regions and cultures. In the case of wine, mezzo- and micro-climates have special needs, and a one-size-fits-all approach (along with the cost) keeps many grape growers from becoming certified.

For now, we have many different organizations setting standards and trying to move agriculture toward lowering the use of toxic chemicals worldwide. Although that is admirable, there's a long way to go in this effort, especially in nonregulated countries, and it can be confusing for eaters and drinkers. Demeter International, for example, has been working at biodynamic certification since 1928, before "organic" existed, and its standards look for the most part to tradition and simplicity rather than innovation and bureaucracy. You hear many farmers say about biodynamics, or about traditional pre-chemical farming, that it's just good farming, and they may be right. But for the moment, especially where certifications are concerned, there's a lot more to it.

The following short discussion of the main certifying bodies may help. This list may not be exhaustive, since new certifications arise every year, but these are the ones I have found on wine bottles and winery websites from the Pacific Northwest region: Washington, Oregon, Idaho, and Northern California, as well as a few in British Columbia. I have organized them from large-scale to small, starting with international and national organizations, down to regional and other groups focusing on education and marketing.

INTERNATIONAL CERTIFICATIONS

The following organizations are based in Europe and have outposts in the United States and elsewhere. Much in the national and regional programs is based on international standards that are constantly being modified. For instance, in 2012, the European Union (EU), through the Standing Committee on Organic Farming (SCOF), tightened its qualifications for "organic" wine, including:

- No desulfuration (or removing sulfur through a mechanical process)
- No sorbic acid added to wine
- Maximum sulfite levels: 100 mg/l (milligrams per liter) for reds, 150 mg/l for dry whites and rosés (50 mg/l lower than before), 30 mg/l for sweeter wines (below the nonorganic maximum)

INTERNATIONAL ORGANIZATION FOR BIOLOGICAL AND INTEGRATED CONTROL (IOBC)

www.iobc-wprs.org

The IOBC, established in 1955, encourages collaboration and education among members (individual scientists, governments, and scientific and commercial organizations) in 24 countries from Europe, the Mediterranean region, and the Middle East. Among other things, it promotes integrated pest management, the use of "environmentally safe, economically feasible, and socially acceptable" pest control for agriculture and forestry. IOBC also carries out studies to develop methods of tracking effects of pesticides and of lowering pesticide use. Certified LIVE members are also internationally certified by the IOBC.

DEMETER CERTIFIED BIODYNAMIC PREPARATIONS

Here are nine certified biodynamic preparations and the claims about their uses:

- BD 500: A cow horn is filled with cow manure and buried on the fall equinox. It is dug up on the spring equinox, and the contents are stirred in water for one hour. The liquid is sprayed on crops to promote microbial life and stimulate root activity.
- BD 501: "Horn silica" is quartzite powder that has been buried inside a cow horn for six months, then mixed with water and sprayed on the leaves and shoots to refract light and stimulate photosynthesis and chlorophyll formation.

These are added to the compost pile:

- BD 502: Yarrow permits plants to attract trace elements.
- BD 503: Chamomile stabilizes nitrogen in the compost and increases soil life.
- BD 504: Nettle stimulates soil health, providing plants with nutrition and enlivening the soil.
- BD 505: Oak bark provides healing qualities to combat disease.
- BD 506: Dandelion stimulates relation between Si (silicon) and K (potassium) to attract cosmic forces to the soil.
- BD 507: Valerian stimulates compost so phosphorus will be properly used.
- BD 508: Horsetail is mixed with water, stirred 20 minutes, and sprayed on vines to prevent or lessen the effects of fungus.

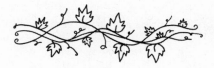

DEMETER CERTIFIED BIODYNAMIC

www.demeter.net

www.demeter-usa.org

The practice of biodynamics began as an agricultural course given in 1924 at Koberwitz, Silesia (now Kobierzyce, Poland), by Austrian philosopher, scientist, scholar, and translator Rudolph Steiner, who also established the Waldorf educational system. The lectures, entitled "Spiritual Foundations for the Renewal of Agriculture," prompted the formation of the Experimental Circle of Anthroposophical Farmers, who began testing Steiner's theories. Demeter International, a certifying organization with a worldwide network of member-inspectors, was established in 1928 and grew throughout Europe. The United States Demeter Association certified its first farm in 1982.

The system demands that the process of farming—including growing grapes and making wines—be completely free of synthetic pesticides, herbicides, rodenticides, and fertilizers. Biodynamics has been called "beyond organics," but it is essentially different in that it aims to manage the entire farm (or vineyard as part of a farm) as a self-sufficient living organism, and to do so in harmony with the natural cycles of the sun, moon, and seasons. There is also a spiritual element, working with what Steiner called the energy and "forms of nature" (the distinct fruit, flower, leaf, and root patterns of various types of plants) to build soil and plant health (although the physical forms of plants and their conversion of sun to energy is as much scientific as spiritual). Cover crops, crop rotation, farm animals, and the presence of natural wildlife are encouraged.

Ideally, each farm works toward complete self-sufficiency in compost, as well as in natural herbal and mineral additives (the "preparations") that are applied to the soil to "enliven" it and the plants' growth and immune systems. These mixtures—especially the one called BD 500, consisting of cow dung packed into a cow horn and buried for months—are said to draw on the spiritual energy of the animals as much as on their natural by-products. They are often purchased from elsewhere, especially for use in areas where their ingredients don't easily grow—Steiner was talking to farmers working in the ecosystem of the European north, not arid southern climates. In the winery specifically, no chemical additives may be added to the wines, and natural yeasts must be used. The certification system is essentially a mentoring process, with new members learning from certified farmer/inspectors. There's much more to this fascinating system and you can find a lot more information about it online.

NATIONAL CERTIFICATIONS

Each country has its own governing body to oversee issues surrounding agriculture and food safety. Much of what these organizations do is in the areas of inspection, safety standards, and communications of allergy alerts and product recalls, as well as establishing labeling standards. To be certified organic, growers must follow certain requirements (including studying the organic standards), comply with approved methods, maintain documentation of their compliance, submit annual production plans that include crop sources, locations, fertilization activity, and more. Each farm must also have an annual on-farm inspection by an independent third-party agency (one of the almost 100 approved by the USDA in the States, for instance). It must pay an annual fee and keep written records on farming and marketing practices in case it is subject to a short-notice or surprise inspection, just as a restaurant may be subject to a surprise inspection from the local health department.

(Unfortunately, there is not room to list all the European certifying agencies here, but a quick internet search will turn up abundant information on the topic.)

CANADIAN FOOD INSPECTION AGENCY (CFIA)

www.inspection.gc.ca

The Canadian equivalent to the USDA, the CFIA uses the European Organic System for certifying organic products. There are two official label designations in Canada: "100 percent organic" means that the wines are produced with 100 percent organically grown grapes, with no sulfur dioxide added; "organic" wines have a minimum of 95 percent organic grapes and low sulfite levels. The phrase "wine made with organic grapes" is now not considered to be an organic designation under the Canadian Organic Products Regulation.

Beyond this labeling issue, Canada does allow EU organic wines to be marketed within the country, as long as they meet Canadian organic guidelines. It also has a country-of-origin labeling program: If a product is "wholly manufactured outside of Canada, the label must show that the product is imported." Wine labels must also include allergens, such as eggs, milk, and other fining agents. The CFIA is currently working toward a better labeling system, as well as stricter regulation of what can be considered ice wine (specifically, that it must be made of grapes frozen naturally on the vine, not in a freezer).

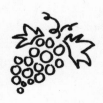

USDA CERTIFIED ORGANIC: NATIONAL ORGANIC PROGRAM (NOP)
www.ams.usda.gov/AMSv1.0/nop

Under the USDA National Organic Program, wineries can become USDA Certified Organic. Here is the official definition:

> *Organic farming is a production system which avoids or largely excludes the use of synthetically compounded fertilizers, pesticides, growth regulators, and livestock feed additives. To the maximum extent feasible, organic farming systems rely on crop rotations, crop residues, animal manures, legumes, green manures, off-farm organic wastes . . . and aspects of biological pest control to maintain soil productivity and tilth, to supply plant nutrients, and to control insects, weeds, and other pests. The concept of soil as a living system is central to this definition.*

USDA Certifications on the Label

USDA certifications provide a wealth of detail on wine labels, specifying whether some or all of the grapes were grown organically and whether or not sulfites were added in the winery. Here is an explanation of the various certifications:

CERTIFIED ORGANIC. For a wine to be labeled organic and bear the USDA organic seal, it must be made from organically grown grapes, meaning no chemical fertilizers, herbicides, or pesticides in the vineyard. Beyond the vineyard, sulfites in the winery are another issue: An organic wine cannot have any added sulfites, apart from naturally occurring sulfites of fewer than 20 parts per million.

MADE WITH ORGANICALLY GROWN GRAPES OR CONTAINS SULFITES. "Made with Organically Grown Grapes" can be used on a label when wineries add sulfur dioxide as an antioxidant, antimicrobial preservative. This is a more common category than Certified Organic, as most people think it is difficult to ship or store a wine without added sulfites, without risking the wine going bad and developing flawed aromas and tastes. Idaho's 3 Horse Ranch, in the Snake River Valley, is a good example of a winery that uses the "Made with Organically Grown Grapes" label. Its estate vineyard is Certified Organic, but its winemakers add the bare minimum amount of sulfites, in order to "ensure stable and delicious wine." If sulfites are added and the total sulfites in the wine are above 10 parts per million, a label must state, "Contains Sulfites."

MADE WITH ORGANIC GRAPES AND MADE WITH ORGANIC AND NON-ORGANIC GRAPES. These labels are rarely used, but if a winery is acquiring grapes from different sources, as many do, it is quite possible that the label may be more common in the future, as people demand more information about the ingredients in their food and wine. If a winery uses grapes from three different vineyards, and only one vineyard is Certified Organic, then it may use the phrase "Some Organic Ingredients" on the label. When this is present, it can be assumed that the grapes came from different vineyards, some organically certified and some not.

SULFITE FREE. According to the Organic Consumers Association, "A wine can make the claim, 'Sulfite Free' or 'No Added Sulfites—Contains Naturally Occurring Sulfites,' but if sulfites are added and the total sulfites in the wine are above 10 parts per million, it must make the statement 'Contains Sulfites.' A wine that makes the claim

Sulfite Free must have no detectable sulfites." It may be impossible to produce a wine with no sulfites at all, as they occur naturally in the fermentation process, but these wines have such low amounts that they are essentially undetectable.

The USDA Certification Process

In order to have a wine certified by an inspecting body, a representative (an actual human being) comes to the vineyard to look it over, and others read the mounds of paperwork the vineyard manager must fill out. At press time, there were 86 USDA-approved certifying agencies across the country. Of these, 28 are approved to inspect farms in California, 9 in Idaho, 19 in Oregon, and 13 in Washington. Oregon Tilth Certified Organic (OTCO) is approved in all these states and is one of the main inspecting agencies for vineyards.

In order to be certified, a vineyard must meet the following conditions:

- It is prohibited from using synthetic substances throughout the year.
- It may use no genetically modified organisms.
- Total sulfites at bottling cannot exceed 100ppm (50 percent less than conventional wines).
- Any additional ingredients, such as sugar, have to be certified organic.
- Products used for cleaning inside the winery cannot be harmful to humans (products like iodine and chlorine are strictly prohibited).
- Any yeast nutrients used during fermentation must contain only organic nitrogen.
- No copper additions can be used in the cellar.

Certifying Agencies for the USDA National Organic Program (NOP)
Of the 86 (and growing) third-party verifying agencies approved
to certify farms as USDA Approved Organic, Oregon Tilth is one
of the largest and can certify in many states. But there are other
agencies across the country that do this work. It is important that
organizations that inspect vineyards not have an economic stake in
the vineyards inspected, to avoid favoritism and ensure objectivity.

California Certified Organic Farmers (CCOF)
www.ccof.org
The California Certified Organic Farmers organization is similar to
Oregon Tilth (see below), certifying farms according to the USDA's
NOP. Founded in 1973, it was one of the pioneers in the certification process. As of the time of this writing, there is a plan to merge
Oregon Tilth and CCOF, to allow the organization to "overcome the
challenges of an uncertain economic future, provide membership
a stronger collective voice, and increase opportunities for all via a
research- and education-focused institutional foundation."

Oregon Tilth Certified Organic (OTCO)
www.tilth.org
Many of Oregon's wineries are USDA Certified Organic through
Oregon Tilth, which has been certifying since 1974. Oregon Tilth
is "an internationally recognized organization of organic farmers,
gardeners, and consumers who are dedicated to biologically sound
and socially equitable agriculture." Its goal is to educate people
about the need to develop and use sustainable growing practices
that promote soil health, conserve natural resources, and prevent
environmental degradation while producing a clean and healthful
food supply.

. . . .

THE GREENWASHING CONTROVERSY

There are some who say that many of these certifications are mostly a reflection of marketing choices, or "greenwashing." A winery may have a small organic vineyard but make the bulk of its wines the conventional way. Another may have an organic vineyard but use copper sulfate for treating fungus in the vineyard or bad-smelling wine in the winery (copper sulfate is allowed under organic certification, but many people call it a "nasty" chemical). Another may make biodynamic wine and sell it in heavy, fuel-hogging bottles that help draw a hefty price. Others can't afford the thousands of dollars it takes to become certified, or simply don't want to pay the money—there's a lot of hassle and paperwork involved. They might wonder whether it is worth their effort and money—especially if they are already farming organically or biodynamically—to have a certification stamp on their label.

In some cases, wine producers choose not to be certified because they would rather be free to do what *they* feel they need to do to keep their specific site healthy. For instance, Klipsun Vineyard, one of *Wine&Spirits* magazine's "25 Great Vineyards of the World," sells fruit to some of the state's top producers, including DeLille and L'Ecole No. 41. Says owner David Gelles, "We've chosen not to be certified by LIVE or Salmon-Safe because of some of the restrictions on some chemicals that we feel we need to use. We haven't used herbicides in 20 years, but there are certain pesticides we periodically need to use." Vineyard manager Julia Wood agrees. "I try to use the softest chemicals, and use them sparingly. Chemicals are expensive!" she says. "We apply them through very precise drip irrigation, and use no organophosphates. We also grow wheatgrass in the rows, which helps to keep the dust down."

An aspect of sustainability that Gelles sees as equally important concerns Klipsun's labor force. It keeps a year-round crew of 14 to 18 workers. "During harvest, we hire the other family members, so the money stays in the family. It allows them to save during harvest, because most of them go south or to Mexico for two to three months." Klipsun also is one of the few vineyards in Washington to provide health care for its employees. "It's easier for a winery than for a vineyard," says co-owner Patricia Gelles, referring to wineries such as Pepper Bridge, which also supplies health care for its employees.

The other side of the argument comes from organic and biodynamic farmers, who say that merely practicing some of these methods while still using Roundup misses the point: Only by giving up the habits of conventional farming and winemaking will the full benefits of organic/biodynamic winegrowing be achieved. Some feel that any certification helps to strengthen the industry and create a positive image, while to others, certification is partly greenwashing and leads the public to believe a wine is more environmentally friendly than it actually may be. Yet still others think that the overall movement toward cleaner wine and a less polluted environment will pay off.

One winegrower who embraced change completely is Doug Tunnell of Brick House Winery, who had been farming organically for 15 years when he transitioned to biodynamics in 2005. This method, he says, has "helped to enliven our soil and integrate our fields, blocks, microsites, gardens, and landscapes into a single living and interdependent whole farm. Compost made up of the remnants of the crush fertilizes our garden and the beds around our house. Leaves from our oak grove help to feed the soil in our vineyard blocks. The result is a vibrancy and life that we didn't enjoy in the years before we practiced biodynamics. And I think our wines are better as a result."

Wine writer Matt Kramer is an advocate of biodynamic wines. "What matters is that biodynamic cultivation signals a willingness to pay extreme attention to vines and wines," he says. "Like driving a race car, if you take your eyes off the road—or in this case, a highly vulnerable vineyard—an irremediable disaster can result. Ask any farmer. Attentiveness is always a good thing."

Whichever direction wine producers take, each change in the vineyard and the winery is a choice not taken lightly, and it is a compliment to this industry that so many conscientious and talented people are growing and making great wine—or letting great wine make itself—and remain willing to wrestle with cultural, environmental, and ethical choices in the production of our beloved beverage.

OTHER REGIONAL PROGRAMS AND MARKETING ORGANIZATIONS FOR SUSTAINABILITY

Salmon-Safe, Fish Friendly Farming, Vinea: The Winegrowers' Sustainable Trust (in Washington's Walla Walla Valley), and Napa Green are grassroots organizations created in response to particular issues in particular regions. They can be points of entry for more strict certifications, such as Certified Organic or Certified Biodynamic. Habitats and ecosystems don't respect state or international borders, though, so many organizations work throughout the larger salmon ecosystem rather than merely in the locale in which they were founded (Oregon, in Salmon-Safe's case). Similarly, Oregon Tilth certifies farms as USDA Certified Organic across the country, and LIVE started in Oregon but looks to be an international organization, recently acknowledged by the IOBC.

Although many of these groups work across borders, it seems simplest to list them here by the state in which their headquarters reside. Some organizations, such as the OCSW, have their own certification stamp (OCSW's means a winery is LIVE and/or Salmon-Safe); this group and others like it work to promote and educate consumers about sustainable products.

CALIFORNIA

CALIFORNIA SUSTAINABLE WINEGROWING ALLIANCE (CCSW, FOR CALIFORNIA CERTIFIED SUSTAINABLE WINEGROWING)

www.sustainablewinegrowing.org

CCSW is a program created by the California Association of Winegrape Growers (CAWG), a trade organization, and the Wine Institute, the marketing arm of California's wine industry. It is a voluntary system of vineyard and winery education and improvement, based on a "Cycle of Continuous Improvement" plan by which winegrowers self-assess, interpret, educate, and develop "action plans" to continually better their vineyard practices. At the time of this writing, there were about 35 participants in the program. It is separate from USDA Organics and aims to improve the California wine industry as a whole. Many states are starting to have certification programs based on wineries' efforts toward sustainability.

From the CCSW website:

> The California Sustainable Winegrowing Alliance (CSWA) developed a third-party certification program related to the California Sustainable Winegrowing Program (SWP) to increase the sustainability of the California wine industry by promoting the adoption of sustainable practices and ensuring continual improvement. The goals of the certification program, Certified California Sustainable Winegrowing (CCSW-Certified), are to enhance transparency, encourage statewide participation, and advance the entire California wine industry toward best practices in environmental stewardship, conservation of natural resources, and socially equitable business practices.

Here is a list of the Alliance's goals:

- Produce the best-quality wine grapes and wine possible.
- Provide leadership in protecting the environment and conserving natural resources.
- Maintain the long-term viability of agricultural lands.
- Support the economic and social well-being of farm and winery employees.
- Respect and communicate with neighbors and community members, and respond to their concerns in a considerate manner.

- Enhance local communities through job creation, supporting local business, and actively working on important community.
- Honor the California wine community's entrepreneurial spirit.
- Support research and education, as well as monitor and evaluate existing practices to expedite continual improvements.

FISH FRIENDLY FARMING (FFF)

www.fishfriendlyfarming.org

Fish Friendly Farming is a certification program for agricultural properties that are managed to restore fish and wildlife habitat and improve water quality. Endangered Coho salmon and steelhead trout are the focus of this California agency, which provides a "voluntary, self-directed compliance with the rigorous standards of state and federal water quality laws (Clean Water Act), the federal Endangered Species Act, and state pesticide laws as well as local regulations."

The Fish Friendly Farming certification "assures the consumer that the wines and farm products they purchase are produced by protecting and restoring the environment and by sustaining the beauty and natural habitats of California." While some vineyards and wineries may struggle to meet the requirements, some go far beyond the standards of organizations such as FFF and Salmon-Safe, depending on the particular situation.

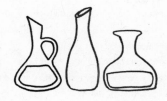

NAPA GREEN (NG)

www.napagreen.org

Through Napa Green, both wineries and vineyards can become certified in a voluntary program (like all of these are) that "enhances the [Napa area] watershed and restores habitat with sustainable agriculture practices," and helps ensure compliance with the Clean Water Act, Endangered Species Act, and state and county conservation laws. Currently, nearly 19,000 acres are certified in the Napa Green Certified Land program, and about 75 wineries have the Napa Green Certified Winery distinction. NG is connected to the Fish Friendly Farming program—to become NGCL, you must also be FFF.

OREGON

CARBON NEUTRAL CHALLENGE (CNC)

www.cncwine.org

In 2007 the Oregon Environmental Council and the Oregon Wine Board joined to lead an initiative to help Oregon wineries and vineyards assess and reduce their carbon footprints, with the ultimate goal of making them carbon neutral. So far, with 14 wineries certified and plans for an additional 16 in the works, this is the largest carbon-reduction effort in the US wine industry. The website describes a three-step process:

1. Calculate the carbon footprint for a winery and/or vineyard operation using a tool based on the Climate Registry's requirements (see www.theclimateregistry.org).

2. Implement a plan to reduce carbon emissions in the winery operations by making smart, cost-effective investments and operational changes; each winery is urged to consider installing renewable energy systems on site. The Oregon

Business Energy Tax Credit, federal tax credits, and Energy Trust incentives provide financial assistance for renewable energy and efficiency upgrades. Energy Trust can support small wind, geothermal, and hydroelectric generating projects. Conversion to biodiesel (B99 or B50) fuel can also reduce emissions. Other investments, such as lighting retrofits, tank insulation, and cellar space portioning, are highly encouraged.

3. Purchase carbon offsets. Wineries can invest in regional and high-quality carbon offset projects located in the Pacific Northwest and managed by the Bonneville Environmental Foundation. The more the carbon footprint is reduced over time, the fewer offsets are required.

FOOD ALLIANCE (FA)
www.foodalliance.org

Food Alliance is an independent, third-party organization created by Oregon State University, the Washington State Department of Agriculture, and the Kellogg Foundation in 1994. It has been certifying farms, ranches, crops, and products according to sustainability standards since 1998, making it one of the most comprehensive nationwide programs. Food Alliance states its mission as follows:

- Protect, conserve, and enhance soil, water, wildlife habitat, and biodiversity.
- Conserve energy, reduce and recycle waste.
- Reduce use of pesticides and other toxic or hazardous materials.
- Maintain transparent and traceable supply chains through record keeping and labeling.
- Support safe and fair working conditions (fair wages, safety compliance).
- Guarantee food product integrity, with no genetically engineered or artificial ingredients.

- Ensure healthy, humane animal treatment.
- Ensure continual improvement of agricultural practices.

LOW INPUT VITICULTURE AND ENOLOGY (LIVE)
www.liveinc.org

Low Input Viticulture and Enology is an Oregon organization that certifies vineyards and wineries in the Northwest (205 in Oregon, 20 in Washington) according to international guidelines for environmental stewardship, social responsibility, and economic accountability. LIVE also provides education and resources to winegrowers interested in sustainable farming. The group was recently endorsed by the IOBC as a qualified certifying body in the United States, and its territory will soon expand to include British Columbia and Idaho.

LIVE's checklists show action areas necessary for certification for vineyards and wineries. For vineyards, these include biodiversity, farm records, traceability, site selection (making sure the site is a viable growing area, performing soil sampling, etc.), grape varieties (determining whether they are the best for the area), rootstock (making sure it is disease-free), sowing, fertilizer use, irrigation, harvesting, post-harvest, animal density, worker health, and more. For wineries: grapes used, energy use, carbon emissions, equipment, sulfur dioxide levels, enology, fermentation, cooling, water management, solid waste, packaging and closures, worker health, facilities, and tasting room issues.

Certified LIVE members are internationally certified by the IOBC. LIVE also works with other organizations, such as Salmon-Safe and Vinewise, a resource for grape growers developed by the Washington Association of Wine Grape Growers to "address the rapidly growing Washington wine industry and to ensure its future." LIVE also administers the Carbon Neutral Challenge program for the Oregon Wine Board and Oregon Environmental Council.

LIVE has a series of regional chairs for each area in the Pacific Northwest: the Willamette Valley (WVTC), Walla Walla (WWTC), Columbia Valley (CVTC), and Southern Oregon (SOTC) Technical Committees. These help determine the needs of each region (pests or climate-related diseases in one region may not be the same as in another), via the Joint Technical Committee.

OREGON CERTIFIED SUSTAINABLE WINE (OCSW)
www.ocsw.org

The Oregon Wine board created OCSW as a marketing body to help "communicate these (sustainable) practices in an understandable manner, highlight shared principles among the various certification philosophies, and forge relationships with consumers who make environmental awareness or action a priority." The OCSW stamp on the label means that at least 97 percent of the fruit used in the wine is certified by an independent third party, such as LIVE, USDA Organic, Demeter Biodynamic, Food Alliance, or Salmon-Safe.

Edward Fus, LIVE Chair Emeritus and owner of Angel Vine Winery and Three Angels Vineyard, says that although the program is small at present, it gives wineries a set of "talking points to help them communicate the sustainable message" to retailers, restaurant staff, and distributors. "LIVE and the other certifiers," he says, "are not set up to promote/educate the public or wine industry about the environmental, economic, and equity elements addressed by certification. OCSW was developed to be a vehicle to achieve this."

SALMON-SAFE (SS)
www.salmonsafe.org; www.salmonsafe.org/bc

Salmon-Safe was founded in 1995 in Portland, to work with farmers and vineyards to prevent erosion and runoff of pesticides into sensitive river and stream habitats for Pacific Northwest salmon and other fish. There are now about 240 certified vineyards across the Pacific Northwest (110 in Oregon, representing a third of Oregon's wine grape acreage). Salmon-Safe is also working with wheat farms, orchards, and dairies to address issues affecting important salmon watersheds upstream in the Yamhill, Tualatin, Walla Walla, Rogue, Columbia, Fraser, and other river basins. The Canadian branch, Salmon-Safe British Columbia, certifies Canadian vineyards in partnership with the Pacific Salmon Foundation (www.psf.ca) and the Fraser Basin Council (www.fraserbasin.bc.ca). Other partners are Oregon's Stewardship Partners and Trout Unlimited.

Oregon Tilth has worked with Salmon-Safe to create a set of additional "overlay" standards for farmers already certified organic. It includes "additional riparian area management, irrigation water use, and erosion control criteria that are either not covered, or are covered only indirectly, under organic certification." A vineyard doesn't have to be certified or even practicing organic to be Salmon-Safe, as long as it meets Salmon-Safe standards applying to pesticides and fertilizers that may create damaging runoff. Some see Salmon-Safe as a first step toward organic certification, since the standards are simpler and less restrictive than for organic. For instance, a vineyard may be near a stream, but the organic certification may not take that into account, focusing only on the crops. Salmon-Safe sees the surrounding areas as important to protect as well, connecting what happens in areas of agriculture to the surrounding ecosystems.

WASHINGTON

VINEA: THE WINEGROWERS' SUSTAINABLE TRUST

www.vineatrust.com

In Washington, some Walla Walla winegrowers, led by Norm McKibben of Pepper Bridge Winery, established their own group tailored to the needs of the Columbia Valley region. Vinea: The Winegrowers' Sustainable Trust is a "voluntary group of winegrowers who have embraced environmentally friendly and socially responsible viticultural practices." The guidelines used are based on those of LIVE, its certifying agency, and the winegrowers work together to promote sustainability in the Columbia Valley AVA, as well as the Walla Walla Valley AVA, which extends into Oregon.

Vinea's mission is to develop a "sustainable vineyard management program that will be internationally recognized for its strict environmental standard and high quality farming and energy conservation practices," including:

- Purchase of renewable energy
- Use of biofuel from recycled vegetable oil for farm vehicles
- Internal energy conservation, through techniques from recycling waste to more efficient tractor usage
- Third-party certification through LIVE
- Registration with the Climate Registry
- Purchase of offsets through the Bonneville Foundation, and local methane digester projects

FOOD AND WINE PAIRING

Traditional wine pairings have often confused me. I *get* red wine with a steak. And white with fish I get—acid with salt, like lemon squeezed on an oyster. But then again, I always eat oysters naked because I like the taste of the oyster and don't want to cover it up with lemon. According to oyster guru Jon Rowley of the Pacific Coast Oyster Wine Competition (www.oysterwine.com), a great oyster wine "cleanses your palate and gets it ready for the next oyster." Some classic pairings, like ruby port with blue cheese, never worked for me. I always preferred figs and nuts with tawny port or a dry sherry. I also felt that cured meat went much better with a lemony white wine than with tannic red. Like a lot of people, after all the advice, I only know what I like. What does this have to do with "natural" winemaking? It turns out (for me), almost everything. Bear with me.

One of the best pairings I've ever had was a moderately buttery, oaky Chardonnay (which I'm not really a fan of) with steak and green peppercorn sauce, thanks to my good friends chef Danielle Custer (then of Seattle Art Museum's Taste Restaurant) and Don Townshend of Townshend Cellars. Danielle has always been thoughtful about pairing; wine and food always go together for her. When she did wine dinners at SAM, she and chef Craig Hetherington would sit down with the wines and with a table full of particular ingredients: beef, lamb, fish, onion, garlic, lemongrass, sage, lemon, whatever. They would taste the wine with each ingredient and then make a menu. The dinners were always amazing. I felt that she got to the essence of what worked with the wines and the specific elements of the ingredients.

When she asked me to come along as she worked with Townshend Cellars' Don Townshend to make a wine for SAM, I jumped at the chance. During our trips to Spokane, we would spend hours tasting and blending different barrel samples, and then cook. Our favorite dish was Don's Green Peppercorn Steak with Townshend Chardonnay. But why did that wine work better than the Cabernet Sauvignon we tried? I didn't know at the time, but now it makes perfect sense.

Green peppercorn has a molecule in it called eugenol, the major molecule in saffron and in a variety of other foods, such as grilled beef and herbs and spices such as rosemary, clove, and basil. The Chardonnay had some of this spicy clove molecule from its time in an oak barrel. At the same time, the sauce had a tiny bit of cream. Lactol is an aromatic molecule in both cream and Chardonnay that has gone through malolactic fermentation (a process that heats the wine and transforms the malic, or appley, acid to lactic, or milky/buttery, acid). It wasn't so much about the meat as about the sauce.

Natural Wines and "Molecular Sommellerie"

I became fascinated with such molecules, including linalool, which is the source of the spicy/floral aroma that you get in Gewürztraminer. But it wasn't until recently that I came across the work of François Chartier, a Québécois sommelier, cook, educator, and writer who wrote the book *Taste Buds and Molecules* (English language edition: Wiley, 2012), which focuses on a new way to pair food and wine, called Molecular Sommellerie. The idea brings together what Danielle Custer was doing—tasting ingredients in their raw form—with what I was learning from Chartier's writing about aroma molecules in food and wine. Yes, like molecular gastronomy, Molecular Sommellerie looks at the building blocks of foods in order to pair them with each other, and with wine. In this case, though, there's no *sous vide* Cabernet foam. The concept is much simpler (and also more complex) than that.

Basically, Chartier says that the main aromatic molecules in all food ingredients, including wine, create an "aromatic synergy" when tasted and smelled together. For instance, Sauvignon Blanc from all over the world has similar flavors of anise, fennel, fenugreek, mint, and "grassiness." Why? Because those all have the molecule sotolone. When Chartier tasted a Sauvignon Blanc along with a simple, fresh tabouleh salad with mint, tarragon, basil, and chervil, he was blown away; the aromas in the wine and the aromas in the food matched, creating a perfect synergy.

He kept experimenting, investigating why some traditional combinations work. For example, he looked at black pepper and Syrah and discovered that both include the molecule rotundone, which gives Syrah its spicy flavor. He eventually worked with amazing "molecular gastronomy" chefs from around the world, including Ferran Adrià from the famous El Bulli restaurant in Spain, pairing wines with foods using this method. Chartier says there's not just one "bitter" but many, not just one kind of acid but many: lemon (ascorbic), apple (malic), milk (lactic), etc. He likens the effect to Shiva, the many-armed goddess: One molecule can have many different manifestations, and most foods have more than one aromatic compound as well as many that are interconnected. Cooking also changes them and brings out even more flavors and even more connections.

Dominant Aroma and Natural Foods

To pair food and wine this way, Chartier suggests, consider the dominant aroma or ingredients in the food and find a wine with the same dominant aroma (or vice versa), to allow the natural aromatic synergy to occur on your palate and in your nose. At the risk of oversimplifying (in hopes that this might spur you on to further reading), here are a few examples:

- Eugenol: Present in various amounts in clove, Thai basil, rosemary, apricot, pineapple, asparagus, grilled and roasted beef, cinnamon, strawberry, and rosemary. It is also found in oak, so a barrel-aged Chardonnay with that clove scent might fit with some of these foods.
- Sotolone: Found in mint, coriander, basil, tarragon, endive, cumin, chervil, and Sauvignon Blanc.
- Rotundone: Found in dried herbs, black pepper, lamb, thyme, cocoa, coffee, citrus, mushrooms, saffron, and Syrah, Grenache, and Grüner Veltliner.
- Linalool: Found in lavender, basil, sweet orange, bay leaf, and Gewürztraminer, Riesling, and Muscat.

So what does all this mean to organic, biodynamic wines? Isn't this too much talk of chemistry for a natural way of eating? To me, it means a lot, because of two things.

First, knowing how these molecules work helps us to understand the flavors we are experiencing in our food and wine. Second, it helps us understand how our experience may be enhanced. These are molecules and compounds that can be isolated and studied by winemakers who want to produce a certain effect in their wines. A 2008 article in the *New York Times* by Harold McGee, "What's the Peppery Note in those Shirazes?," talked about Australian studies on rotundone in 2002 and 2003 that found that timing of harvest and time on the skins (where this molecule lives) affect the amount of pepperiness in the wine. It would be illegal to add rotundone to wine to create a desired effect, but other methods, such as filtering or clonal selection, can reduce overpepperiness in wine and can make a big difference. The wine industry goes to great lengths to find out what works and what doesn't.

Also, if you are reading this book, you may be interested in enjoying "natural" foods and wines together and experiencing their purest nature. If you are the type who's willing to pass by those bright-red tomatoes in the produce section, knowing that they'll taste like cardboard, and wait until August for true tomato flavor, then you probably want the same from your wine. A naturally made wine, with the least manipulation, chemical additives, commercial yeasts, etc., allows the flavors and aromas of the fruit and natural yeasts to shine through, making for a more authentic—and delicious—experience.

. . . .

OTHER CERTIFICATIONS TO LOOK FOR

These are just a few of the many other organizations that support and promote sustainable winegrowing and winemaking.

BEE FRIENDLY FARMING (BFF)

www.pfspbees.org

The Partners for Sustainable Pollination are based in Santa Rosa, California, and have a "self-certification" process to help beekeepers, orchardists, vineyards, and others manage their farms and products in the interest of protecting and creating bee-friendly habitat. Certification allows producers to use the BFF logo on their products. There are almost 200 BFF farmers in 31 states and 3 provinces of Canada, but only one winery—Jordan Vineyards in Healdsburg, California.

LEADERS IN ENERGY AND ENVIRONMENTAL DESIGN (LEED)

www.usgbc.org

The United States Green Building Council (USGBC) is an independent international nonprofit that sets standards for environmentally friendly construction and energy and water usage. LEED is an arm of the USGBC and is a professional membership organization made up of 77 chapters, 13,000 member organizations, and 181,000 LEED professionals—builders and environmentalists, corporations and nonprofits, teachers and students, lawmakers and citizens. More and more, wineries and tasting rooms are building green and receiving certifications at different levels, from Silver to Gold to Platinum.

THE LODI RULES FOR SUSTAINABLE WINEGROWING CERTIFIED GREEN (LR)

www.lodiwine.com

The Lodi Rules, established in 2005 but based on the work of the Lodi, California, winegrowing community going back to 1992, was California's first third-party-certified sustainable winegrowing program, promoting biodiversity, soil and water health, and community and employee well-being, with more than 21,000 acres certified.

RAINFOREST ALLIANCE FOREST STEWARDSHIP COUNCIL (FSC)

www.rainforest-alliance.org

The FSC certifies all sorts of products from wood to cardboard packaging to corks (and many others, such as eco-friendly shampoo and cleaners). It favors conservation of the cork forests over the use of screwtops or plastic corks (see the "Put a Cork in It" sidebar).

SONOMA COUNTY WINEGRAPE COMMISSION (SCWC)

www.sonomawinegrape.org

The SCWC is just one example of the dozens of commissions in winegrowing regions that support their industries. More and more, the focus among these folks has been, How do we make winegrowing more sustainable environmentally and as an industry? Each area has taken its own approach (Lodi Rules; Napa Green; Mendocino, "America's Greenest Wine Region"), with programs and websites that promote the wineries of the area. More than 390 grape growers in Sonoma County were involved in a California-wide self-assessment Code of Sustainable Winegrowing study in 2002, which was part of a statewide Sustainability Report, confirming their vineyards to be "environmentally sound, socially equitable, and economically viable." The SCWC helps provide ongoing assessment and education for this large and vital grower community.

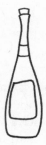

A State-by-State Guide to Green Winemaking

It used to be that if you wanted information about a winery's sustainable practices, you had to call and hope the winemaker wasn't in the middle of washing out tanks. Now the information is available on websites; there's often a tab marked "Sustainability" or "Organics." Sometimes the story or certification information is up front, sometimes it is hard to find. (I would urge wineries to list any certifications somewhere on their websites.) Nothing replaces a visit to a vineyard or a face-to-face chat with a winemaker, of course, and the list that follows is the product of a combination of vineyard and winery visits, interviews, conversations, and online and print research. Information on this subject is always changing, and while this list can't provide every detail about every sustainable winery, it offers a sturdy starting point for your own explorations.

Is the move to say as much in promotional materials about carbon neutrality and raptor poles as about fermentation and aging just a marketing trend? To some, perhaps. But the more you talk to people who are farming organically, even with biodynamic techniques (certified or not), the more passionate talk you hear about how their vineyards, their soil, their wines—and their lives—have improved as they have become increasingly committed to sustainable farming and natural winemaking. Not just in the vineyard anymore, sustainability is about energy conservation, solar and other renewable sources, efficient and recycled construction, and shrinking the winery's overall carbon footprint. And whether all this is done to save money, to save the planet, or merely for marketing's sake, well, that may or may not matter. It is a move in the right direction, and away from destructive practices espoused by the majority of large conventional farming and viticultural operations. There's a long way to go, but as consumers, we need to ask questions and educate ourselves on the facts behind the wines. In the process, we'll forge stronger connections with winegrowers and winemakers.

This book is just a first foray into this vast subject, and for the sake of educating the consumer (and myself) I've chosen to present a broad array of growers and producers from all sides of the issue. The selection of wineries that follows—in Northern California, Oregon, and Washington, with a few in Idaho and British Columbia—should provide a good overview of what various producers are doing in the area of sustainability as a whole. There are of course many more incredible individuals, vineyards, and wineries out there (and growing in number every day) focused on making the best wine they can in a sustainable manner. I hope to visit them all eventually, to learn about their ways and pass on their stories. In the meantime, the wineries listed here all contribute to the overall picture. On your next visit to a wine grower, maker, or purveyor, I encourage you to further flesh out that picture with questions of your own.

WINE BY-PRODUCTS: VERJUS

The "nose to tail" culinary movement of recent years revived old-fashioned recipes using often-ignored parts of hogs, cows, and even chickens. Heart, tripe, liver, sweetbreads, and trotters are now on the menu at many American restaurants. A similar trend is emerging in the wine world, what you might call the "whole grape" movement. In traditional winegrowing societies, by-products of the harvesting and winemaking process were used in various ways, from composting pomace (seeds, skins, stems, and pulp left over from crush) to the production of grappa, a distilled spirit. Another by-product, verjus (*vehr-ZHOO*), is common in Europe and the Middle East (called *husroum* in Arabic and *ab-ghooreh* in Persian) but is just starting to show up on gourmet food shop shelves in the United States. In ancient Rome it was called *acresta* (*agresta* in modern-day Italian) and used to marinate meats. In Syria, the tradition of producing husroum brings women together for several days to press grapes and distribute the tart liquid to farflung family members. In northern France, crabapples are used to make verjus as well.

Verjus (from the Middle French *vertjus*, or "green juice") is the non-alcoholic, unfermented juice of unripe red or white grapes. It has a sweet-tart flavor, due to the fact that the grapes are picked just as they begin to ripen. Often winegrowers will do "green pruning"—pruning off fruit when the grapes are green—to drop a certain percentage of the crop to increase the intensity of flavor and ripeness of the remaining grapes. These grapes are left on the ground to decompose back into the soil, or are added to compost, but that is a shame, since verjus is not only delicious but can pull a high price at specialty food stores. At Klipsun Vineyards on Red Mountain in Washington, winegrowers Patricia and David Gelles and their son Alexander have been producing a vintage verjus since 2003, harvesting

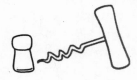

the grapes in July and bottling them at local wineries. Fusion, a Napa Valley verjus producer, exposes the juice to heat for just four seconds to purify it, then uses aseptic packaging, which preserves the verjus and keeps it from fermenting spontaneously, without the use of chemicals.

Whether made from red or white grapes, verjus can be used in myriad ways for drinking and cooking, as you would use vinegar, lemon juice, or wine. It can deglaze the brown bits in the bottom of a pan to start a sauce, and makes a lovely salad dressing. I drink it over ice, in a cocktail, use it for marinades, and to brighten up soups. It's good for any sauce that needs a bit of zing, such as beurre blanc, and for white sauces for fish, and is heavenly when mixed with melted duck fat and drizzled over sautéed chard or kale.

Several wineries make and sell verjus, and since these are vineyards that either don't use any chemicals or use them only rarely for focused problems, you can count on these brands to be as pure as possible:

- Alexander the Grape / Klipsun Vineyards Verjus, 500 mL, $20
- Abacela Verjus, 750 mL, $15
- Bonny Doon Verjus de Cigare, 750 mL, $10
- Fusion Napa Valley Verjus, 750 mL, $10
- Montinore Estate Biodynamic Verjus, 750 mL, $20
- Navarro Vineyards, 750 mL, $7.50
- Seufert Winery, 750 mL, $15
- Trium Wines Baby Bacchus Verjus, 750 mL, $19.95
- Venturi-Schulze, 375 mL, $12

HOW TO USE THIS GUIDE

The abbreviations listed below represent the various certifications described in the Certifications section of this book. Keep in mind that certifications are constantly changing, being renewed, added, or let go by a vineyard or winery for a whole host of reasons. All wineries have tasting rooms unless otherwise indicated. Furthermore, not all wines from a particular winery may be organic or LIVE-certified, so look for icons on the back of the bottle or ask your wine producer. (A certification applying only to particular wines will be followed by the names of those wines, in parentheses.)

Finally, note that this list is by no means exhaustive; it is only a sampling of the possible certifications out there, and there are other small regional and organization certifications that may not have made it to these pages. Complete, up-to-date lists of certified wines, wineries, and vineyards can usually be found on the websites of each organization.

I suggest "Wines to Try" throughout the listings. These are wines that I have come across and enjoyed, and I hope you will, too.

INTERNATIONAL

DB   Demeter Certified Biodynamic (International)

UNITED STATES

CCOF   California Certified Organic Farmers (certifying agent for USDA)

CO   US Department of Agriculture Certified Organic National Organic Program

FA   Food Alliance

OTCO   Oregon Tilth Certified Organic (certifying agent for USDA, Oregon and other states)

REGIONAL

CCSW   California Certified Sustainable Winegrowing

DRC   Deep Roots Coalition (Oregon)

FFF   Fish Friendly Farming (California)

LIVE   Low Input Viticulture and Enology (Oregon, Washington, California, Idaho, and British Columbia)

NGCL   Napa Green Certified Land

NGCW   Napa Green Certified Winery

OCSW   Oregon Certified Sustainable Wine (usually means both
LIVE and Salmon-Safe)

SS   Salmon-Safe (Oregon and international)

VINEA   Vinea: The Winegrowers' Sustainable Trust (Washington,
based on LIVE)

ENERGY AND PACKAGING

BFF   Partners for Sustainable Pollination's Bee Friendly Farming
(California and other states, Canada)

CNC   Carbon Neutral Challenge (Oregon Wine Board and Oregon
Environmental Council)

FSC   Rainforest Alliance Forest Stewardship Council (international:
packaging, cork)

LEED   US Green Building Council's Leadership in Energy and
Environmental Design

· ·

RANDALL GRAHM: 13 WAYS OF LOOKING AT A WINE LIST

It's been a bit of a rocky road for Bonny Doon Vineyards owner and wine-maker Randall Grahm, but not only in the way you might think. Grahm has embraced the mystical side of winemaking, and it's not just the practice of biodynamics, which he has advocated for years. In fact, he finds the unknown a big part of why he loves wine. Take, for instance, "minerality," a subject of much debate and not a lot of hard fact (no pun intended). It is detected in the aromas, flavor, and mouthfeel of wines, in elements described as "stony," "chalky," "flinty," or "earthy." The wine list at his now-defunct Le Cigare Volant Restaurant—the organic restaurant that was part of Grahm's small winery in the warehouse district of Santa Cruz, Cali-fornia—featured, in addition to all the Bonny Doon wines (some Demeter certified), a fascinating assortment of Grahm's favorite wines from around the world, focusing on minerality instead of fruitiness. Where a "taste profile" wine list (the one I put together at the Doe Bay Café on Orcas Island in the San Juan Islands of Washington State, for instance) might categorize wines by fruit profile (Red Fruits and Bright Acidity, for example, or Big, Bold, and Black Fruit), the categories in Grahm's list have more to do with rocks: flinty, gravel, volcanic, granite, etc.

It is a whole different way of looking at wine. But then, Grahm has a whole different way of looking at wine in general. He started Bonny Doon Vineyard in 1983, producing until his vineyard was tragically destroyed by Pierce's disease in 1994. After that, he bought grapes from other California vineyards, blending them into delicious, inexpensive, interesting wines that took off in the American market. His Big House Red, Big House White, and Cardinal Zin were some of the first to bring a sense of humor to the wine market. He sold those brands (and most of his other labels) in 2006 and started Pacific Rim, a Riesling-only winery in Washington State, the same year. Grahm produced 10 different food-friendly Riesling wines, from bone dry to sweet, and the company acquired what is now Wallula Vineyard in the Wallula Gap area near Walla Walla. He sold the project in 2011 and now has only his small Bonny Doon Vineyard winery, mostly purchasing grapes from biodynamic vineyards in northern California but also growing fruit in his own dry-farmed Ca' del Solo Vineyard in Monterey County.

Grahm's Le Cigare Volant wines get their name from the fact that in 1954, Châteauneuf-du-Pape banned "les cigares volant"—flying saucers—from landing in its vineyards after a series of UFO sightings in France. Right up Grahm's *allée*, the old-fashioned Max Ernst–esque collage label features a blimp shining its light onto the vineyards of unsuspecting vignerons. The wines are grown biodynamically and are beautifully aromatic, especially the Ca' del Solo Estate Nebbiolo, which is like an Italian Pinot Noir, with bright cherry fruit but, more importantly, a stoniness that makes it memorable. Wine scientists haven't determined where this minerality comes from, whether it is influenced by the soil the grapes grow in, or from a variety of elements that result in a lack of fruitiness in the wine, creating an impression of a mineral element. Grahm has gone as far as conducting experiments by adding ground-up rocks—rip rap (granite), Noyo, cobble stone, black slate, and Pami pebbles—to wine to see how it changes the flavor and texture.

Whatever the reason, Grahm is fascinated by wines that show this expression of terroir. He sees winemaking as a collaboration. It includes, of course, himself and the other people working in the winery, but the focus is on the fruit and the sun, and "the yeasts themselves must be the primary suspects, vis-à-vis, 'winemakers,' but at a minimum, we can propose that 'winemaking' is somewhat of a group effort." The collection of elements that contribute to Grahm's wines—and the discussion and amusement that surround them—should only grow in interest as we continue to enjoy fascinating wines made by this pioneer of natural wine.

NORTHERN CALIFORNIA WINERIES

> *California is starting to dial back on the power and brawn, picking grapes at lower sugar levels and concentrating on matching the grape varietal with the soil type. Finally, California wine is emerging from the id stage to embrace its superego. In other words, as a wine region, the state is starting to grow up.*
>
> —Alice Feiring, author of *Naked Wine: Letting Grapes Do What Comes Naturally*

California has always been a leader in organics, since long before the first hippies left the cities to start communal farms and get "back to the land." Winegrowers there have been pioneers too, because wine grapes are a sensitive fruit and require attention that many other agricultural crops do not. Of course, California is a huge state—of mind. There are as many styles of farming as there are farms. It may be impossible to capture the range of stories and the gamut of sustainable practices in the state, even among the most dedicated wineries, but I have tried to sample from a range of wineries, vineyards, and approaches from all parts of Northern California and a few farther south. Some have been farming organically for decades, some planted biodynamic vineyards just a few years ago; some are massive wineries, some are minuscule. But all have similar goals: to make delicious wines, while taking better care of the land, the water, the air, and the people around them.

AMBYTH ESTATE
DB
510 Sequoia Lane · Templeton, CA 93465
(805) 305-9497 · www.ambythestate.com

AmByth is the Welsh word for "forever," and winegrowers Phillip Hart and Mary Morwood Hart are committed not only to biodynamic farming but to 100 percent dry farming, meaning no irrigation is used in the vineyards. They also practice natural winemaking, relying on natural yeasts on the grapes and in the air for fermentation, adding no outside chemicals to manipulate the wines, and not filtering or fining the wines to make them more clear. "Biodynamic farming not only encourages the elimination of all chemicals," says Hart, "but encourages the farmer to pay close attention to the forces of nature influencing his/her farm entity." Of this 42-acre property, only 20 acres are planted in vineyards; the other 22 are left as natural woodlands and fields, to encourage a diverse population, including the farm animals, bees, olive trees, fruit and nut trees, and vegetable gardens. The Harts landscape with native and edible plants, with "minimal-to-zero" water usage.

ARAUJO ESTATE WINES

DB · FFF · NGCL · NGCW
2155 Pickett Road · Calistoga, CA 94515
(707) 942-6061 · www.araujoestate.com

Bart and Daphne Araujo, owners of the century-old Eisele Vineyard, have created wines with cult status by hiring the top people in the business to guide them through the process. Winemaker Tony Soter (formerly of Spottswoode Estate Vineyard and Winery and others; now at Soter Vineyards in Oregon) was their first consulting winemaker, and world-famous French consultant Michel Rolland stops in periodically, consulting on the biodynamic winemaking process. But the estate, set in a riparian valley on a dry creek bed at the foot of Calistoga's Saddleback Mountains, is also a functioning farm with hundreds of century-old olive trees, honeybees, vegetable gardens, plus cows and chickens that wander the fields. These all are a part of the whole-farm philosophy of biodynamics, using everything on the farm—animal waste, compost, beneficial insects—to support what grows there. Director of winemaking Françoise Peschon and winemaker Nigel Kinsman produce exquisite wines at prices that suggest a "money is no object" approach. They usually produce four wines each year: Cabernet Sauvignon Eisele Vineyard; Altagracia (which includes grapes from other vineyards, farmed to their specifications); Syrah Eisele Vineyard; and Sauvignon Blanc Eisele Vineyard. Some years they add a Viognier, also from the Eisele Vineyard.

BARRA OF MENDOCINO

CO
7051 N. State Street · Redwood Valley, CA 95470
(707) 485-0322 · www.barraofmendocino.com

Eighty-four-year-old Charlie Barra likes to say of his 175-acre organic vineyard in Redwood Valley, "I've really been farming organically for 50 years . . . I just didn't know it for the first 30!" A third-generation farmer, he now grows Pinot Noir, Zinfandel, Cabernet Sauvignon, Sangiovese, Merlot, Petite Sirah, Chardonnay, Pinot Blanc, Pinot Grigio, and Muscat Canelli. He sold his grapes to organic wineries such as Beringer and Fetzer for years before starting the Barra of Mendocino label in 1997. In 2001, his wife, Martha, realized that they would probably do well to focus on Pinot Noir as well, so they created the Girasole label. Wine-maker Jason Welch follows organic practices in the winery. Wine writer Patrick Comiskey notes, "Their Pinot Noir, about $15, is as well priced for what's in the bottle as any in California."

BEAVER CREEK VINEYARDS
CCOF · CO · DB
22000 California Highway 29 · Middletown, CA 95461
(707) 987-1069 · www.beavercreekvineyards.com

Beaver Creek Vineyards, north of Calistoga in Lake County, is a collab-oration between Czech-born winegrowers/winemakers Martin Pohl and Radan Bruno Kolias, and partner Josef Rusnak. To Pohl's way of thinking, biodynamics is not a method but a way to "bring nature back into bal-ance. It is a direction that is one step beyond organic which we use to create an outstanding, original wine that is an expression of harmony between vines and winemaker." Their farm teems with animals: Chick-ens, goats, rams, and cows wander the vineyards and do their part to keep the weeds at bay. The horns used to make biodynamic preparation #500 come from their own cows. They also use small amounts of sulfites, only when needed to preserve the wines and protect against oxidation.

BENZIGER FAMILY WINERY
DB   ·
1883 London Ranch Road · Glen Ellen, CA 95442
(888) 490-2739 · www.benziger.com

Benziger was one of the first wineries to go biodynamic, when Mike Benziger saw that his soil was getting "harder and drier and quieter." In the mid-1990s, Mike consulted with his friend Alan York, who happened to be an international biodynamics expert, and, before it was a common thing at all—in France, let alone in California—converted all four of the estate vineyards to biodynamics. When you visit Benziger and take the 45-minute Biodynamic Vineyard Tram Tour, you get the full treatment: a ride in a golf-cart-like bus, a tour of the property and caves, and a primer on biodynamics. This is a unique property, positioned in an extinct volcano caldera 800 feet above sea level. The folks at Benziger feel that biodynamics helps make the most of this place, because it is a "closed system": Recycling all the agricultural waste back into the property in order to build the soil and plant health helps create wines that reflect this special site.

Wines to Try: Benziger's Tribute wine is a different blend each year, usually of Cabernet Sauvignon, Cabernet Franc, and Malbec. This wine is made to highlight the biodynamic process in the vineyard and minimal processing in the winery, letting the grapes express their truest nature without excessive manipulation.

BONNY DOON VINEYARD
DB
328 Ingalls Street · Santa Cruz, CA 95060
(831) 425-4518 · www.bonnydoonvineyard.com

The poet-philosopher (and, of course, cult winemaker) Randall Grahm has been a proponent of biodynamic winegrowing for years and has followed these practices in the Ca' del Solo Vineyard exclusively since 2004. Grahm makes the distinction, as the French do, between wine that is *vin de terroir* (referring to wines of a place) or *vin d'effort* (wines made in the winery, more manipulated by the winemaker). When he started out, he purchased grapes from many vineyards, as many wineries do, and therefore had to do more manipulation in the winery to ensure a consistent product. But since he has taken control of the wine-growing process, purchasing some grapes from vineyards he respects, and focusing on letting his vineyard nourish and enliven itself through composting and spraying herbal and compost preparations onto the plants, he has been making wines "the old-fangled way," with much less manipulation in the winery, allowing the grapes to express the site and the process of their growth in the wine.

Wines to Try: The Cigare Volant series are beautiful, aromatic wines, best enjoyed in their eponymous home-away-from-homeland, Le Cigare Volant tasting room connected to the winery in Santa Cruz.

BONTERRA ORGANIC VINEYARDS
CCSW · CO · DB · FFF
2231 McNab Ranch Road · Ukiah, CA 95482
(800) 846-8637 · www.bonterra.com

Mendocino is the center for organic viticulture in California, and Bonterra Vineyards is a leader, with 900 certified organic and biodynamic acres that produce beautiful wines. Bonterra's McNab Ranch, Butler Ranch, and the Heron's Reach (home to 20 great blue herons that nest in the trees each year) are gorgeous, unique vineyards with beautiful gardens full of flowers and herbs attracting bees and other beneficial insects. A huge old barn has been converted to a tasting room. McNab Ranch is located in a box canyon with high hills all around a deep valley, where daytime temperatures can be over 100°F and nights are very cool and foggy, creating conditions that allow Pinot Noir grapes to develop incredible character and acidity. Over the years, vineyard director Dave Koball and lead winemaker Robert Blue have planted each block to highlight the aspect, climate, and soils of this special site. Instead of a marketing coordinator, this winery has its own "Organic Life Aficionado," Lia Huber, to help spread the word of the benefits of the organic life.

Wines to Try: The Muscat is an explosion of honeysuckle, apricot, peach, and lime zest and truly tastes like a pure expression of beautiful fruit.

BUCKLIN
CCOF · CO
8 Old Hill Ranch Road · Glen Ellen, California 95442
(707) 933-1726 · www.buckzin.com

The 14-acre Old Hill vineyard, planted by William McPherson Hill in 1880, is one of the oldest blocks in the New World and is planted with mostly Zinfandel interplanted with Alicante Bouschet, Petite Sirah, Mourvèdre, Syrah, Carignan, Tempranillo, and a dozen other varieties. Although the yields are super low, about 1.5 tons per acre, the wine output is growing into an amazingly delicious and complex history lesson in a glass. The newest owners—the four siblings Arden, Kate, Ted, and Will, the children of Otto and Anne Teller—bought the vineyard next door to their grandmother's vegetable and flower farm in 1981 and started a winery in 2000. They are no longer just selling grapes to other wineries, as their parents did. USDA Certified Organic, the now-60-acre Old Hill Ranch is also dry-farmed, and some of the wines are made as "field" blends, an Old World style of making wine from various types of grapes growing in the same vineyard, rather than planting blocks of one variety, as is the norm today. When the Tellers bought the property, this vineyard was overgrown and unrecognizable, but Ravenswood winery's Joel Peterson offered to buy the fruit if they revived the vines. In 1983, Ravenswood Old Hill Zinfandel was released, and 30 years later the vines are producing the complex Bucklin Old Hill Ranch Zinfandel. Farmed much the same as it was in 1880, the farm has come full circle, sustaining a family over generations.

CEAGO VINEGARDEN
DB
5115 California Highway 20 · Nice, CA 95464
(707) 274-1462 · www.ceago.com

Ceago (from a Pomo native word for "grass-seed valley") is more than just a vineyard and winery. Owner Jim Fetzer, former head of one of the first and largest organic wine producers in California, started this project in 1993. It includes 163 acres on Clear Lake in Lake County, and the original 132-acre "Camp Masut," in Mendocino County. It produces an array of excellent biodynamically and organically grown wines and conducts a whole lineup of "Biodynamic Estate" and "Farm-to-Table" tours as well. Fetzer has embraced the whole-farm approach of biodynamics, growing various vegetables and fruits on the property, as well as herbs, kiwis, olives, walnuts, and lavender. There are also 40 Rambouillet sheep, which help keep weeds and grass controlled and are a source of meat and beautiful wool. Dozens of Rhode Island Red chickens wander the vineyards, eating cutworms that can feed on vine roots and supplying the staff with fresh eggs. Like other biodynamic farms, Ceago composts intensely and applies biodynamic preparations such as BD 500 and 501 to foster growth, photosynthesis, and overall plant health.

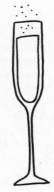

• •

MENDOCINO VINO: AMERICA'S GREENEST WINE REGION

Mendocino County is becoming known as the most sustainable winegrowing region in California. A collection of 10 AVAs, Mendocino County is the umbrella AVA, with the Mendocino AVA overarching six other, smaller AVAs: Anderson Valley, Yorkville Highlands, McDowell Valley, Potter Valley, Redwood Valley, and America's smallest AVA, Cole Ranch. Each region has unique characteristics, from the rugged hills of Anderson Valley to the hot daytime temperatures of Potter Valley to the cool, misty hillsides of Mendocino Ridge. Of the 20,000 acres planted, 28 percent are certified organic, which is 400 percent more acreage than in any other US wine region.

Frey Vineyards in Mendocino was one of the first certified-organic vineyards, joining CCOF in 1980. It produced the first wine in the country to be made from certified-organic grapes. Now Mendocino County has 343 growers and 91 wineries, including 10 Demeter Certified Biodynamic wineries, 21 with certifications for organic, and another 8 using organic practices but not certified. Other wineries, such as McDowell Valley Vineyards, went solar before any others in the country, and Parducci was the first carbon-neutral winery in the United States. Fetzer generates more solar energy than any other winery in the United States, with 1.1 million kilowatts powering its buildings.

All this reflects the roots of Mendocino culture, with its origins in the hippie movement of the 1960s and its many farmers who came to the area to get away from the city. For Mendocino wine, it has been a long road that has paid off in a vital, enthusiastic collection of wineries producing some of the best—and greenest—wines in the country.

• •

DAVERO
DB
766 Westside Road · Healdsburg, CA 95448
(707) 431-8000 ext. 3 · www.davero.com · By appointment only

Since 1982, Ridgely Evers and Colleen McGlynn have modeled their farm on the farms they loved on visits to Tuscany. It just so happens that this model dovetails nicely with biodynamics, encouraging the integration of diverse crops and animals and fostering biodiversity. DaVero (Italian for "Indeed!" or "the real thing") grows much more than grapes: The farm is filled with olive trees (from which they make and sell oil), Meyer lemons, oranges, tangerines, peaches, plums, apples, pears, blackberries, quinces, figs, persimmons, pomegranates, lavender, and tons of vegetables. Ridgely and Colleen keep chickens for eggs and also raise pigs. From their 16 acres of Dry Creek/Russian River vineyards, they produce a Sangiovese, a red blend, a rosé of Sangiovese, and a fascinating Sagrantino (an Italian grape with bright-red fruit and rose-petal aromas). You can book a tour of the vineyard with groups of 4 to 12 people and be part of their Tuscan dream.

DELOACH VINEYARDS
DB
1791 Olivet Road · Santa Rosa, CA 95401
(707) 526-9111 · www.deloachvineyards.com

DeLoach Vineyards' story is classic California. Established in 1973 by Cecil DeLoach, a firefighter from San Francisco with a passion for winemaking, the winery became known and much lauded for its Pinot Noir. In 2003, Jean-Charles Boisset of Boisset Family Estates in Burgundy, France, the ancestral home of Pinot Noir, fell in love with the site and purchased the winery. Boisset is a leader in sustainable winegrowing and winemaking, one of the first to use Tetra Pak alternative packaging in his French Rabbit wines. Boisset converted DeLoach to biodynamic farming, following the lead of most of the Burgundy region, and in 2010 the first biodynamic and organic wines were produced—a seven-year wait, showing how the wine business must think ahead, and also must wait, for good wine. It is easy to see why sustainability is becoming a watchword for this changing industry, since, more and more, it is essential to look toward the future of wine.

Wines to Try: DeLoach's Estate Pinot Noir is a good wine to start with, made from its first certified-biodynamic harvest in the cool 2010 vintage, with full plum and raspberry fruit balanced with baking spice and earth, and fermented with native yeast.

PAUL DOLAN VINEYARDS / MENDOCINO WINE COMPANY
CCOF · CCSW · CO · DB
501 Parducci Road · Ukiah, CA 95482
(888) 362-9463 · www.pauldolanwine.com

Part of the Mendocino Wine Company—a partnership between brothers Tim and Tom Thornhill that also owns Parducci Wine Cellars (see listing below), Sketchbook Wines, Wines That Rock, and Zig Zag Zin—Paul Dolan Vineyards is near Parducci and focuses on biodynamics as a way to create premium wines of the highest quality. Dexter cows and Araucana chickens wander fields of California poppy, where bees buzz and pollinate. Although Paul Dolan himself, a leader in biodynamic and organic winegrowing, is not connected to the Paul Dolan brand anymore, he continues to grow grapes in other vineyards and is looking to start a new brand. Tom and Tim Thornhill will continue to farm Paul Dolan Vineyards wines biodynamically, which is in line with how their other wineries are managed.

Wines to Try: A good choice is Filligreen, a 100 percent organic Pinot Noir grown in the Anderson Valley and Mendocino County AVAs. It has a bright red cherry and earth nose with a soft vanilla finish from its time spent aging on French oak.

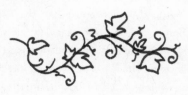

EHLERS ESTATE

DB

3222 Ehlers Lane · St. Helena, CA 94574

(707) 963-5972 · www.ehlersestate.com

The Ehlers Estate vineyard has been growing grapes since as far back as the mid-1800s, when Bernard Ehler established it. Owner Jean Leducq acquired this and surrounding vineyards, replanted them, and by 2001 began making wine to honor the farm's history. He died in 2002, and the vineyard was left to the Leducq Foundation, which he and his wife founded in 1996 to benefit international cardiovascular research. Now, 100 percent of the wine profits goes to the Leducq Foundation. The vineyards have been biodynamically farmed since 2005, and winemaker and general manager Kevin Morrisey feels that the "intimate, hands-on attention given at every stage of winegrowing" makes this vineyard special. The Cabernet Sauvignon, Merlot, Cabernet Franc, Petit Verdot, and Sauvignon Blanc blocks are managed by a full-time, seven-person vineyard crew that passes through the 25 different sub-blocks many times. As the season nears, they pass through to drop fruit six times or so, in order to ensure the health and quality of the remaining fruit. That's a lot of work, but it creates a more focused, elegant wine free of unripe flavors and with all the complexity the fruit can develop.

FETZER

CCSW · CO · FFF

Hopland, CA

www.fetzer.com

No tasting room

Since 1968, the Fetzer family—Barney and Kathleen (who died in 1981 and 2010, respectively) and their 11 children—have steered their winery in the direction of sustainable winemaking; the kids worked in the vineyard with Charlie Barra after school, learning organic practices. They created the Bonterra brand in 1990, which focused on organic—and now biodynamic—wines. In 1992, the Fetzers sold the Fetzer Vineyard brand to Brown-Forman Corporation, which built up the brand as an "earth-friendly wine." Brown-Forman also improved the winery's infrastructure, constructing a 10,000-square-foot rammed-earth administration office building, using almost exclusively recycled materials. It has one of the industry's largest solar arrays, at 899 kilowatts and was the first to use 100 percent renewable energy. It has reduced companywide waste 96 percent since 1990, from 1,724 tons to 65 tons in 2010. In 2005, Dr. Ann Thrupp, Fetzer's manager of organic development, became the managing director of the Wine Institute's California Sustainability Winegrowing Alliance, which creates standards for wineries across the state. After growing the Fetzer brand—which included closing the much-loved tasting room and inn in Mendocino—Brown-Forman sold it to Chile's Viña Concha y Toro for $238 million. Which raises important questions: Can this type of huge growth occur without affecting sustainability? If organic falls out of fashion, will the company's commitment to it waver? Viña Concha y Toro has many other brands focusing on sustainability and bought Fetzer partially because of the "green" direction it had established. But will the company be a leader in the movement, or is it merely following a trend it hopes will pay off? At any rate, the very consistent, well-made wines are worth trying, and are available across the country in many more places than those of smaller, "green" wineries.

Wines to Try: Fetzer wines are some of the most available and accessible sustainably produced wines, and the variety is broad, from refreshing Pinot Grigio from Mendocino to deep, rich Malbec from Mendoza (although this has more wine miles, for sure). The wines I have enjoyed most are the light whites; a moderately oaked Chardonnay with melon, soft citrus, and vanilla-spice notes is a lovely all-around table wine.

FREEMARK ABBEY
DB

3022 St. Helena Highway N. · St. Helena, CA 94574
(800) 963.9698, ext. 3721 · www.freemarkabbey.com

The people at Freemark Abbey have been forward thinkers since 1886, when Josephine Tychson became one of the first woman winegrowers in California, opening up her winery along Highway 29, where Freemark Abbey now stands. Built in 1899, the stone building was never really an abbey; the name dates to 1939 and is actually a combination of those of the three owners at the time: Charles Freeman, Markquand Foster, and Albert "Abbey" Ahern. Although Freemark has several vineyards scattered across Napa Valley, one of them, Sycamore Vineyard, is special, in that it is farmed biodynamically. It is a cooler-climate vineyard set up against the Mayacamas Range, where the Cabernet Sauvignon thrives without irrigation, producing tiny, intensely aromatic fruit. All of Freemark's wines are noteworthy, but this Cab is exceptional (and priced so, at $100 a bottle).

FREY VINEYARDS
DB

14000 Tomki Road · Redwood Valley, CA 95470
(707) 485-5177 · www.freywine.com

If biodynamics is the "It takes a village" approach to winegrowing, then Frey is its Royal Family. The oldest certified-organic winery in the country, and the first producer of a Demeter Certified Biodynamic wine in the country, Frey Vineyards, in the Northern Mendocino AVA of Redwood Valley, was ahead of its time. Since the 1960s, it has eschewed herbicides and other chemicals, composted, and utilized "green manure," or cover crops of grasses, legumes, and mustards that create habitat for beneficial insects, prevent erosion, and fix nitrogen in the soil. Now, Mendocino boasts the largest acreage of certified-organic vineyards in the United States, and Frey has consulted for many vineyards that have followed the organic path. The family is a large one, led by Paul and Marguerite "Beba" Frey, two doctors who met in New York City, moved to Mendocino in the 1960s, and had 12 children. That would seem like enough work for a lifetime, but their passion for farming and wine has kept the family farm going strong ever since. The concept of the biodynamic farm as a self-sustaining unit lives up to its fullest potential with this family: All 12 children, and now their children, have a role to play, whether it is Paul Frey Jr. as president and winemaker, or Luke Frey as biodynamics expert, or Adam Frey, the mechanical whiz kid who maintains equipment on the farm, to daughters Karla (an osteopath) and Julia (a mother and writer), who set up key accounts to grow the winery.

FROG'S LEAP WINERY
CO · FFF
8815 Conn Creek Road · Rutherford, CA 94573
(800) 959-4704 · www.frogsleap.com

Owner John Williams's mantra is "Reduce, reuse, recycle, renew, retain, and revere," and Frog's Leap has tried to apply that prescription in every aspect of the business. The vineyard is not irrigated and has been farmed organically since 1988, planted in cover crops like crimson clover, vetch, Austrian winter pea, and oats to help build the soil and encourage good bugs to live in the vineyard in order to deal with bad bugs. Owl boxes bring nighttime flyers to keep the rodent population down. Frog's Leap wines are excellent, reflecting a commitment to purity, and, like many other wineries in sunny California, it has shifted toward solar energy, with 1,020 photovoltaic panels on a half acre of vineyard space, supplying 100 percent of its energy needs and sending the excess to Pacific Gas & Electric. Over the 30-year lifetime of the panels, they will reduce fossil fuel emissions by 1,600 tons (like planting 450 acres of trees, or not driving 4 million miles). Although the project was pricey at $1.2 million, with a PG&E rebate of 50 percent the system pays for itself in six years.

Wines to Try: One of Frog's Leap's most popular and widely available wines is its Sauvignon Blanc, a light, refreshing wine with flavors of grapefruit, peaches, and lemon zest.

GRGICH HILLS ESTATE
DB
1829 St. Helena Highway · Rutherford, CA 94573
(800) 532-3057 · www.grgich.com

Mike Grgich has lived the quintessential American Dream. Born Miljenko Grgic in Croatia in 1923, he studied enology at the University of Zagreb in 1949 and ended up in Napa—with a new Americanized name. Grgich worked, among other places, at Beaulieu Vineyards with André Tchelistcheff, a pioneer in the wine industry, and had the good fortune to become the winemaker at Napa's Chateau Montelena—now famous in the movie *Bottle Shock*—where his 1973 Chardonnay beat out the French at the 1976 "Paris Tasting." In 1977 he established his own vineyard, and he now owns a total of 366 acres, planted in five vineyards in American Canyon, Carneros, Yountville, Rutherford, and Calistoga. His grand-nephew Ivo Jeramaz joined the winery in 1986 and eventually took over winegrowing and winemaking duties from the now 90-year-old patriarch. But the dream has been taken to its next level, building on the traditional farming practices that Grgich has always followed to now farm all 366 acres biodynamically, making Grgich Hills the largest Demeter Certified Biodynamic farm in the country.

Wines to Try: Grgich Hills makes classic California Zinfandel grown in their Calistoga vineyard with no artificial fertilizer, pesticides, or herbicides. This is a Zinfandel-lover's Zin, with deep, rich strawberry fruit and licorice, spice, and pepper.

HAWK AND HORSE VINEYARDS
CCOF · CO · DB
13048 California Highway 29 · Lower Lake, CA 95457
(707) 942-4600 · www.hawkandhorsevineyards.com

Mitch and Tracey Hawkins and Tracey's stepdad, David Boies, and his family are farming 18 acres of a 1,300-acre estate in the Red Hills AVA of Lake County and have been certified biodynamic since 2008 and CCOF certified organic since 2004. Mitch manages the vineyard, and Tracey, along with consulting winemaker Dr. Richard Peterson, makes the wine, but the ranch was really the vision of Boies, who envisioned creating world-class wine and purchased this historic property in 1999. Once the home of El Roble Grande, California's largest valley oak (estimated to be 500–800 years old), which came down in a storm in 1952, the ranch is now home to Scottish Highland cattle, who help with composting, and all sorts of wildlife, including wild turkeys, deer, mountain lions, and numerous birds. The tasting room has a ranch feel, displaying tack and saddles from the ranch's history, and Mitch and Tracey lead tours of the property, talking about its history and telling of their adventures in biodynamics.

LA CLARINE FARM
Not certified
Somerset, CA
(530) 306-3608 · www.laclarinefarm.com
No tasting room

La Clarine is a fascinating case study in the journey to natural wine-making. Caroline Hoel and Hank Beckmeyer had farmed their 10-acre, 2,600-foot-elevation vineyard in the Sierra foothills organically since 2001, growing a field blend of Tempranillo, Syrah, Tannat, Grenache, Negroamaro, and Cabernet Sauvignon (as well as purchasing organic grapes for some wines), until Hank came to feel that most philosophies of farming, whether conventional (of course), or even organic and bio-dynamic, are about trying to control the vineyard too much. So he stepped back and asked, "What would happen if the farmer played more of the role of caretaker than active participant? What if much of what we were doing to our land and plants was really not necessary, done more for our own human benefit (ego) than for the benefit of the plant? What if we stepped back and just watched?" So he did, and he has come to the conclusion that a noninterventionist philosophy—what the Japanese farmer/philosopher Masanobu Fukuoka, author of *The One-Straw Revolution* called, essentially, "do nothing" farming—works for him, in his particular vineyard. In the winery, he vowed not to add anything to the wine that would "alter its chemistry or speed fermentation or flavor. The new wine is simply allowed to be what it is at its own pace." As he admits, giving up that control can be scary, but he feels that the wines have the time and tools to develop incredible complexity through this process.

LITTORAI WINES
FFF
788 Gold Ridge Road · Sebastopol, CA 95472
(707) 823-9586 · www.littorai.com
By appointment only

Ted and Heidi Lemon's farm is "modeled on Rudolf Steiner's vision of an integrated farm." Ted worked in France as a winemaker for years and then in California, becoming one of the most in-demand winemakers in the country and also becoming convinced of the benefits of sustainable winegrowing. He sources grapes from selected vineyards all over the state, which he carefully oversees, but he also has a 30-acre farm in Sonoma County, 8 acres of which are fields and streams and 14 acres are pastures for the cows and hay. Part is sown with legumes, grains, and grasses for green manure; the Lemons are reestablishing native grasslands on 3 acres, removing invasive species. Three acres are a Pinot Noir vineyard, and the winery is a straw-bale building, which is energy efficient, not to mention beautiful, with a gravity-flow system to eliminate the need to pump the delicate Pinot Noir grapes. Since Littorai is not certified biodynamic by Demeter, the Lemons don't use that term. In fact, they have decided not to become certified in any of the systems, because they believe that "the true motivation for engaging in sustainable farming practices should not be for marketing purposes but should be only for the good of the land, for the good of those who work it, and for the future generations to whom it truly belongs."

PARDUCCI WINE CELLARS / MENDOCINO WINE COMPANY
CCSW · DB · FFF
501 Parducci Road · Ukiah, CA 95482
(707) 462-9463 · www.parducci.com

Parducci Wine Cellars is Mendocino County's oldest winery, established in 1932, and is now the heart of Mendocino Wine Company. Parducci calls itself "America's Greenest Winery" and applies sustainable practices to every aspect of its business, right down to the soy-based ink on the labels. Parducci was the first carbon-neutral winery in the United States, working with the California Climate Action Registry to calculate annual greenhouse gas emissions, then mitigate those emissions through means like using biodiesel in vehicles and heating and cooling the winery with 100 percent renewable power (using its own solar panels and purchasing Green-e-certified wind energy). Parducci's energy savings are equivalent to taking 66 homes off the grid or taking 87 cars off the road for a year. But even with all this talk of energy, the vineyards are still the focus. They are farmed biodynamically and organically. Owner and green visionary Tim Thornhill, who is focused on making Mendocino County a completely sustainable winegrowing region, says, "I see sustainability as an evolution; we can always find room for improvement."

Wines to Try: Parducci True Grit Reserve wines are small-lot wines from select vineyards in the Mendocino appellation. The 100 percent estate-grown Grenache is a great food wine, with bright, ripe raspberry and pepper notes.

PUMA SPRINGS VINEYARDS
DB
Healdsburg, CA
www.pumasprings.com
No tasting room

Tony Crabb and Barbara Grasseschi bought a slightly neglected vineyard between the Alexander and Dry Creek Valleys near Healdsburg and immediately set out to convert it to a biodynamic farm. They introduced permanent cover crops between the rows to attract ladybugs and bees, built birdhouses to attract insect-eating swallows, and created perching areas for rodent-hunting raptors. They employ a small army of goats to manage unruly weeds and grasses. Tony and Barbara see the biodiversity of the farm as being essential to the life and health of the vines, and the quality of the wines. Puma Springs is part of the Benziger "Farming for Flavors" program, supplying sustainably grown grapes for its wines.

Wines to Try: The grapes for the 2005 Benziger Cabernet Sauvignon were grown in Tony and Barbara's Puma Springs vineyard and are full of dark fruits, tobacco, and tea aromas. Intensely structured with firm tannins, this is a great food wine. Only available online or at the Benziger winery tasting room (see listing above).

QUIVIRA VINEYARDS & WINERY
DB · FFF
4900 W. Dry Creek Road · Healdsburg, CA 95448
(707) 431-8333 · www.quivirawine.com

Sixteenth-century maps of the Sonoma area show the mythical gold-paved kingdom of Quivira, and to proprietors Pete and Terri Kight—who bought the vineyard from the first owners, Henry and Holly Wendt, in 2006—their grapes are their gold. Ninety-three acres over several vineyard sites across the Dry Creek AVA in the northern coastal area of California are farmed in a variety of ways, from basic avoidance of chemical herbicides to full-on Demeter biodynamic certification. Winemaker Hugh Chappelle and assistant winegrower Ned Horton bring a wealth of knowledge to their roles, which include "chicken rancher," with several different breeds inhabiting their "chicken condo," including Black Frizzle Cochins, Cuckoo Marans, Partridge Rocks, and Silver Laced Wyandottes. Energywise, Quivera uses 100 percent solar to power the property's buildings, and a steam barrel-cleaning system lowers water usage by 98 percent. It is currently working on restoring Wine Creek, the stream that runs through the property, to enhance Coho salmon and steelhead trout spawning grounds. Known for Zinfandel and Sauvignon Blanc, Quivira increasingly produces Rhône-style wines from Grenache and Syrah and Mourvèdre, all using indigenous yeast and minimal sulfites.

SHAFER VINEYARDS
Not certified
6154 Silverado Trail · Napa, CA 94558
(707) 944-2877 · www.schafervineyards.com
By appointment only

Doug Shafer went through what many winegrowers experienced when transitioning to sustainable farming over the past 20 years. His father,

John Shafer, had established 210 acres of vineyard and produced excellent wines in 1978, and when Doug took over as winemaker in 1983, the vineyards looked perfect, with not a blade of grass, not a weed, not an insect in sight. But he knew that was not the direction the vineyard should be going; he started composting, planting cover crops between the rows, and encouraging songbirds and bats to be his "eating machines" to take care of the blue-green sharpshooters and leafhoppers. Perch poles attract red-shouldered hawks, red-tailed hawks, and American kestrels, so rodent poisons are not needed to stop gophers and moles eating young vine roots. "Between the hawks and owls," says Doug, "we have day and night rodent patrol." He also has had bat boxes designed by wildlife consultant Greg Tartarian of Wildlife Research Associates in Petaluma, and hopes to increase the flying-hunter population. Shafer Vineyards now uses 100 percent solar energy, selling its extra back to the utility company for credits. Its wines have long been admired, and Doug hopes the "future farming" practices will increase the quality of the wines and ensure that the vineyard is around for a long time.

ROBERT SINSKEY VINEYARDS
CCOF · CO · DB · FFF
6320 Silverado Trail · Napa, CA 94558
(707) 944-9090 · www.robertsinskey.com

Over the last 25 years, father and son team Robert and Rob Sinskey have transformed a passion for wine that began with a small family winery into a much-lauded operation with 200 acres of organic and biodynamic-certified vineyards in the super-pricey Stag's Leap and Carneros areas of Napa Valley. Rob Sinskey's not a winemaker, but he hires the best, and his luscious Pinot Noirs have attracted fans around the world. When he took over his father's operations in 1981, he adopted a new mantra, "Let the vineyards do the winemaking," and began feeding the fields with compost, cover crops, biodynamic preparations, and more compost. What resulted is a collection of luxurious, elegant Pinot, Cabernet Sauvignon, Cabernet Franc, Merlot, Pinot Gris, and Pinot Blanc. At Sinskey, the marriage of wine and food is literal, as Rob's wife, former chef Maria Helm Sinskey, is "chief cook and bottle washer" for the on-site professional kitchen, the Vineyard Kitchen. She cooks up wine-friendly bites, and posts recipes and a gallery of instructional images on the website.

OTHER CALIFORNIA WINERIES WITH GREEN CONSIDERATIONS

Here are a few more out of the hundreds of California wineries (now there are 3,000-plus total in the state) getting into the sustainable game. I am constantly discovering new wineries that observe various practices or hold various certifications. Make your own discoveries by looking at labels, checking websites, and asking your wine purveyor. Better yet, take a road trip (in an electric car) to visit some of these amazing wineries and see for yourself!

AMPELOS CELLARS
312 N. 9th Street
Lompoc, CA 93436
(805) 736-9957
www.ampeloscellars.com
DB

BECKMEN VINEYARDS
2670 Ontiveros Road
Los Olivos, CA 93441
(805) 688-8664
www.beckmenvineyards.com
DB (Purisima Mountain Vineyard)

BJORNSTAD CELLARS
Sebastopol, CA
(888) 356-7696
www.bjornstadcellars.com
No tasting room

BLACK SEARS ESTATE WINES
2615 Summit Lake Drive
Angwin, CA 94508
(707) 965-9650
www.blacksears.com
CO

BYBEE VINEYARDS & HABITAT
9499 Mill Station Road
Sebastopol, CA 95472
(707) 823-9001
www.bpinot.com
Some biodynamic practices

CERITAS WINES
3379 Cerritos Avenue
Los Alamitos
Orange, CA 90720
www.ceritaswines.com
DB (Porter-Bass Vineyard)

COTURRI WINERY
6725 Enterprise Road
Glen Ellen, CA 95442
(707) 525-9126
www.coturriwinery.com
CO

DONKEY & GOAT
1340 5th Street
Berkeley, CA 94710
(510) 868-9174
www.donkeyandgoat.com
Natural winemaking

DUMOL
11 El Sereno
Orinda, CA 94563
(925) 254-8922
www.dumol.com
FFF (Estate vineyard)

ELIZABETH SPENCER WINES
1165 Rutherford Road
Rutherford, CA 94573
www.elizabethspencerwines.com
DB

HEIBEL RANCH VINEYARDS
1241 Adams Street, #1043
St. Helena, CA 94574
(707) 968-9289
www.heibelranch.com
CO

HOBO WINE COMPANY
8437 Grape Avenue
Forestville, CA 95436
(707) 887-0833
www.hobowines.com
DB (Beasley Vineyard)

JERIKO ESTATE (Daniel Fetzer)
12141 Hewlitt and Sturtevan Road
Hopland, CA 95449
(707) 744-1140
www.jerikoestate.com
DB · FFF

JORDAN VINEYARDS &
WINERY
1474 Alexander Valley Road
Healdsburg, CA 95448
(800) 654-1213
www.jordanwinery.com
BFF

KAMEN ESTATE WINES
111B E. Napa Street
Sonoma, CA 95476
(707) 938-7292
www.kamenwines.com
CO

LONG MEADOW RANCH
WINERY
738 Main Street
St. Helena, CA 94574
(707) 963-9181
www.longmeadowranch.com
CO · FFF

LUTEA WINE CELLARS
Santa Rosa, CA
(707) 592-0568
www.luteawinecellars.com
No tasting room
DB

MABOROSHI WINE ESTATES
Sebastopol, CA
www.maboroshiwine.com
No tasting room
DB

MASÚT VINEYARD &
WINERY
1301 Reeves Canyon Road
Redwood Valley, CA 95470
(707) 485-5466
www.masut.com
CO

MONTEMAGGIORE
2355 W. Dry Creek Road
Healdsburg, CA 95448
(707) 433-9499
www.montemaggiore.com
DB

NARROW GATE VINEYARDS
4282 Pleasant Valley Road
Placerville, CA 95667
(530) 644-6201
www.narrowgatevineyards.com
DB

PATIANNA ORGANIC
VINEYARDS
Hopland, CA
(707) 744-8706
www.patianna.com
No tasting room
CO · DB · FFF

PORTER-BASS WINERY
11750 Mays Canyon Road
Guerneville, CA 95446
(707) 869-1475
www.porterbass.com
DB

PORTER CREEK VINEYARDS
8735 Westside Road
Healdsburg, CA 95448
(707) 433-6321
www.portercreekvineyards.com
DB

PRESTON VINEYARDS
9282 W. Dry Creek Road
Healdsburg, CA 95448
(707) 433-3372
www.prestonvineyards.com
CCOF · CO · FFF
Some biodynamic practices

QUINTESSA
1601 Silverado Trail
St. Helena, CA 94574
(707) 967-1601
www.quintessa.com
FFF
Biodynamic practices, working
on certification

RADIO-COTEAU
Forestville, CA
(707) 823-2578
www.radiocoteau.com
No tasting room
DB

RAYMOND VINEYARDS
849 Zinfandel Lane
St. Helena, CA 94574
(707) 963-3141
www.raymondvineyards.com
By appointment only
DB

TOPEL WINERY
125 Matheson Street
Healdsburg, CA 95448
(707) 433-4115
www.topelwines.com
Some biodynamic practices

TRUETT HURST
5610 Dry Creek Road
Healdsburg, CA 95448
(707) 433-9545
www.truetthurst.com
DB

UNTI VINEYARDS
4202 Dry Creek Road
Healdsburg, CA 95448
(707) 433-5590
www.untivineyards.com
Some biodynamic practices

VERGE
Healdsburg, CA
(707) 490-4585
www.vergewine.com
No tasting room
Organic with some
biodynamic grapes

VIADER
1120 Deer Park Road
Deer Park, CA 94576
(707) 963-3816
www.viader.com
By appointment only
Some biodynamic practices

VML WINERY
4035 Westside Road
Healdsburg, CA 95448
(707) 431-4404
www.vmlwine.com
DB

WILD HOG VINEYARD
Cazadero, CA
(707) 847-3687
www.wildhogvineyard.com
No tasting room
CO

YORKVILLE CELLARS
25701 Highway 128
Yorkville, CA 95494
(707) 894-9177
www.yorkvillecellars.com
CO · FFF

OREGON WINERIES

Oregon came later to the certification game than California, but vineyards in Oregon have had the "pure wine" mindset since the beginning. Among the first growers here were winemaker Richard Sommer, who planted Riesling in the Umpqua Valley in 1961 and established Hillcrest Vineyards, and David Lett, who moved to Oregon in 1965 "with 3,000 grapevines and a theory" and planted Pinot Noir, Chardonnay, Pinot Gris, and a few other grapes in 1966, producing his first wine, the Eyrie Vineyards Pinot Noir, in 1970. Lett went on to win the admiration of wine lovers from around the world and helped establish Oregon as a serious Pinot Noir growing region.

Lett, Sommer, Charles Coury, Dick Erath, and others who came to Oregon during that time, as well as those who put down roots a decade later—David and Ginny Adelsheim, Ronald and Marjorie Vuylsteke, Richard and Nancy Ponzi, Joe and Pat Campbell, and Bill

Blosser and Susan Sokol Blosser, and others—were inspired by the great wines of Burgundy and found the climate of the Willamette Valley conducive to growing these delicate and persnickety grapes. Since Pinot Noir takes such care—growers must spend more time one-on-one with their vines, and the grapes are more sensitive to heat, rain, and frost—it makes sense that organics were the way to go. The use of harsh chemical herbicides or pesticides seems at odds with the sensitive and delicate nature of Pinot. In the last 20 years, with more than 300 wineries and growing, Oregon has made sustainability a watchword, not for marketing purposes only (although it does help consumers to know how the grapes are grown), but because these practices work for Oregon, both for the wine and for those who live among the vines.

A TO Z WINEWORKS / REX HILL VINEYARDS
CO · DB · OCSW · SS (Rex Hill Vineyards: estate and single vineyard wines)
P.O. Box 489 · Dundee, OR 97115
(503) 554-1918 · www.atozwineworks.com · www.rexhill.com

Owners Bill and Deb Hatcher have created a winery that sells great Pinot Noir and Pinot Gris for great prices. Their crack winemaking team of Sam Tanahill and Cheryl Francis has an impressive pedigree: working at Oregon's premium Archery Summit and Chehalem wineries for eight years. Now they blend wines from different vineyards to create balanced, dynamic, delicious—and affordable—wines. They believe in the screwtop as a way to avoid cork failure and avoid the chemicals used in cork production. They source from dozens of vineyards around Oregon, all certified organic and biodynamic as well as LIVE and Salmon-Safe, and are one of the 14 wineries participating in Oregon's Carbon Neutral Challenge, to shrink their carbon footprint. In

2007, A to Z bought Rex Hill Winery, a premium Pinot Noir producer, whose Jacob Hart and Pearl Vineyards became Demeter Certified Bio-dynamic in 2008.

Wines to Try: A to Z's wines are consistently excellent, but my favorite is its delightful Chardonnay, which has no oak and is a great example of why Oregon Chardonnay is attracting so much attention lately. "Bright acidity, with aromas of white blossoms, pears, lime zest, and almonds" is a common description of this consistently bright and balanced wine, which is usually blended from several different lots.

ABACELA
SS · LIVE
12500 Lookingglass Road · Roseburg, OR 97471
(541) 679-6642 · www.abacela.com

Abacela is one of Oregon's most distinctive wineries. Focusing on Spanish varietals such as Albariño and Tempranillo, which flourish in the warmer climate of southern Oregon, winemaker Earl Jones has received many awards and converted many fans to these unique wines. In addition to lovely, aromatic, varietally correct whites, reds, and rosé, the winery also produces verjus. Its port-style wines are also much lauded and are made from the five traditional port varieties—Tempranillo, Tinta Amarela, Bastardo, Tinta Cão, and Touriga Naçional—grown in Jones's Fault Line Vineyard. LIVE and Salmon-Safe certified, Abacela is also committed to the Carbon Neutral Challenge; among other measures, Abacela uses perhaps the most-renewable energy source, gravity, to move its grapes from the picking bin to the destemmer, fermenter, and press. "The must is created naturally, albeit very slowly, by using the yeast's fermentative process to soften and eventually 'liquefy' the fruit." This process saves the energy and effort of moving grapes around by machine or hand and is much gentler on the grapes as well.

Wines to Try: Abacela is one of the few producers of the Spanish Albariño grape in the United States. Full of peach and soft citrus aromas, this wine is delicious with fresh oysters and wine-steamed clams.

ADELSHEIM VINEYARD
LIVE · OCSW · SS (estate and single vineyard wines)
16800 N.E. Calkins Lane · Newberg, OR 97132
(503) 538-3652 · www.adelsheim.com

One of the oldest wineries in Oregon, Adelsheim has been a leader in putting Oregon wine on the map, since owners David and Ginny Adelsheim planted their original vineyard in 1972. In recent years it has also gotten on board with Oregon's efforts to lower the environmental impact of the wine industry. With the development of LIVE in the Willamette Valley, Adelsheim has been more and more involved in sustainability practices, lowering its use of chemicals in the vineyard and shifting packaging to recycled and lower-weight bottles. Each Adelsheim wine bottle currently weighs 3 ounces less than earlier bottles. As a result, each truckload of wine is 2,600 pounds lighter than in previous years, so more wine can fit on a truck and less fuel is used in shipping.

Wines to Try: Adelsheim Pinot Noir is classic Oregon, with lush red fruits, minerality, and balanced structure. I'm drawn to the Auxerrois, an eccentric, little-known Alsatian grape well-suited to Oregon's cool climate. The wine is beautifully balanced with acidity and pear and orange blossom, and even herbal notes such as fennel and tarragon.

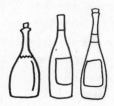

AMITY VINEYARDS
LIVE · OCSW · SS (estate and reserve wines)
18150 S.E. Amity Vineyards Road · Amity, OR 97101
(503) 835-2362 · www.amityvineyards.com

Myron Redford has been making wine at Amity for 40 years, and in his time he's seen a lot of changes. He was an early proponent of organic farming and founding member of the LIVE program, and now his winery, like so many others, is promoting its sustainable practices as an added benefit for the consumer who wants "clean" wine and cares about the environment. Amity offers three certified organic wines without sulfites: Eco Pinot Blanc, Eco Marechal Foch, and Eco Pinot Noir. Redford says that many of the current sustainable practices are win-win. "The sustainable practice in many cases not only improves the environment, but can save money," he says. For instance, he stopped using herbicides and stopped tilling up weeds, and started using a low-impact cover crop. "Once the investment is made, you save money every year."

ANAM CARA CELLARS
LIVE · OCSW
306 N. Main Street · Newberg, OR 97132 (on Highway 240)
(503) 537-9150 · www.anamcaracellars.com

Husband and wife team Nick and Sheila Nicholas established the first 27 acres of Pinot Noir, Gewürztraminer, and Riesling in the Chehalem Mountains AVA in 2001, and a further 6 acres of Riesling, Chardonnay, and Wädenswil Pinot Noir were planted in 2008, this time according to the biodynamic calendar. Part of the original plum, hazelnut, and walnut orchard on the property still stands, and apple, cherry, quince, and pear trees invite beneficial insects to the beautiful fields. After a two-year certification process involving inspection of the vineyards and winery, Anam Cara became LIVE certified in 2010.

Wines to Try: The Nicholas Estate Vineyard Pinot Noir is usually aged in older oak for a lighter style, with red fruits, mineral and herbal notes of bay and camphor, and a lovely floral aroma.

ANNE AMIE VINEYARDS
LIVE · OCSW · SS (estate wines)
6580 N.E. Mineral Springs Road · Carlton, OR 97111
(503) 864-2991 · www.anneamie.com

Anne Amie Vineyards, in the Yamhill-Carlton AVA, is owned by businessman and philanthropist Dr. Robert Pamplin, who works with winemaker Thomas Houseman and vineyard manager Jason Tosch. "It's all about building momentum until sustainability is no longer a selling point," said Thomas Houseman in an interview for Oregon Certified Sustainable Wine. "I would love for us to do to the wine world what Alice Waters has done for food—help build awareness of how your choices affect the larger picture." He feels that choices made by consumers will help drive the market toward a higher level of sustainability on the production end. "It's not just about buying the cheapest 'this and that' but thinking about how that purchase affects the future health of the planet," he says. "Wouldn't it be great if commercial farming eventually became the odd man out?"

ARGYLE WINERY
LIVE · OCSW
691 N. Highway 99W · Dundee, OR 97115
(503) 538-8520 · www.argylewinery.com

The inimitable Rollin Soles, a long, tall Texan (and longtime Oregonian) whose passion for bubbles has been a boon to us all, believes that Oregon's burgeoning sparkling-wine industry is a great match for the climate. "In years that we can't ripen Pinot Noir and Chardonnay grapes, we can still make excellent sparkling wine," he says. Grapes for sparkling wine are picked earlier than grapes for other wines. Argyle sources grapes from three vineyards—Knudsen, Stoller, and Lone Star—that are farmed according to LIVE and Salmon-Safe practices, reducing if not eliminating the use of chemicals in the vineyard. Soles also uses biodiesel in his vehicles, and uses 97 percent recycled-content shipping boxes and inserts from West Coast Paper Co., made in Corvallis, Oregon, from Eugene's *Register-Guard* newspaper. Perhaps all the good reviews of Argyle's wines written in newspapers adds something to the "compost" that feeds this dynamic business.

Wines to Try: Although best known for its sparkling wines, Argyle's Pinot Noir and Chardonnays are both worth noting. Its Nuthouse Chardonnay is juicy and bright, with flavors of white peach and sweet spice, along with a note of toasted hazelnut.

BENTON-LANE VINEYARD
23924 Territorial Highway · Monroe, OR 97456
(541) 847-5792 · www.benton-lane.com
Proprietary program

After seven years of certification with LIVE, Benton-Lane decided to combine various parts of the sustainable, organic, and biodynamic methods into a "Proprietary Program for Care of the Land" that it feels works better for its vineyard. For instance, organics allows copper sulfate, which many people feel is a harsh chemical. "We believe it is better for our land to use soft fungicides like Elevate, with a soil half-life of only one day instead of the organic recommendation of toxic copper," says owner Steve Girard. In the vineyard, the winegrowers also use grazing sheep to keep weeds and grasses under control, a practice that some sustainable certifications don't support. Benton-Lane composts all its grape skins, seeds, and stems, peppermint, rock dust, manure, and estate soil together to spread on the vineyards, and uses mineral oils for pesticide control. It also has kept a large part of the land as a buffer; surrounding the 138-acre vineyard are 175 acres of woods, full of native plants, which serve as a habitat for wildlife and attract beneficial insects.

BETHEL HEIGHTS VINEYARD
LIVE · OCSW
6060 Bethel Heights Road N.W. · Salem, OR 97304
(503) 581-2262 · www.bethelheights.com

In 1977, Ted Casteel, Patricia Dudley, Terry Casteel, and Marilyn Webb, together with Patricia's sister Barbara Dudley, bought property 75 acres north of Salem in the Eola Hills, and now this second-generation operation is enjoying its 35th year of growing grapes. The winery was established in 1984, and owner Marilyn Webb says, "Coming to the Willamette Valley to grow grapes and make wine seemed like the ultimate extension of gardening: growing grapes and then 'putting them up' in the most elegant way." Vineyard manager Ted Casteel was one of the founding committee members of the LIVE program, helping to set standards for sustainable certification, working toward raising standards for agriculture across the whole Oregon wine industry, and giving consumers a way to gauge that commitment. Bethel Heights has been certified LIVE since 1999. It also gets 40 percent of its energy through solar power, with a 60-kilowatt solar panel system that was installed in 2010.

Wines to Try: Bethel Heights has bottled several vineyard-designated wines from individual sites on the property. Look for Pinot Noirs marked Southeast Block, Flat Block, West Block, and Justice Vineyard.

BERGSTRÖM WINES / DE LANCELLOTTI FAMILY VINEYARDS
DB
18215 N.E. Calkins Lane · Newberg, OR 97132
(503) 554.0468 · www.bergstromwines.com · www.delancellottifamily
vineyards.com

John and Karen Bergström wanted to create a farm that "pays tribute to John's Swedish farming heritage," so they planted their Bergström Vineyard in the spring of 1999. No chemicals have been used on this vineyard in more than a dozen years, and the landscape encompasses oak forests full of mushrooms, islands of grasses, insect-attracting flowers, and herbs such as chamomile, which is used in one of the eight biodynamic preparations (made into a tea and sprayed on the vine leaves, to help protect them from disease). Now the Bergströms farm a total of 84 acres in five vineyard sites: The Bergström Vineyard, de Lancellotti Family Vineyards, the Winery Block, Gregory Ranch, and Le Pré du Col. The Bergströms' son, Josh, went to France to study viticulture and enology, and now he and his wife, Caroline, are at the center of the Bergström wine world, farming biodynamically and finding admirers of their unique, pure wines.

Paul and Kendall (née Bergström) de Lancellotti also farm biodynamically and share a winery with Bergström Winery; Kendall, the daughter of John and Karen Bergström, is working with her winemaker husband to develop this new winery as a part of a growing winemaking family. These wines are made to the same exacting standards as Bergström's, using the best of Burgundy's Pinot Noirs as a model.

Wines to Try: Bergström Pinot Noirs are among Oregon Pinot Noir royalty; try the de Lancellotti Vineyard Pinot, and give it a good long while to open up and reveal its complexity and purity of fruit.

BISHOP CREEK CELLARS at Urban Wine Works
LIVE · SS

1315 N.E. Fremont Street · Portland, OR 97212
(503) 493-1366 · www.bishopcreekcellars.com

Bishop Creek Cellars keeps things down to earth. Most of the older Pinot Noir on the 15 acres of vineyard (on a 60-acre site) is planted on its own roots, not grafted onto phylloxera-resistant rootstock, like most vines in much of the world. While, on the one hand, this makes the plants more vulnerable, winemaker Jeremy Saville feels that it makes the wines taste better and express their Pinot Noir-ness "from root tip to shoot tip." Bishop Creek works to eliminate erosion by creating a wide buffer zone around streams and wetlands on the property, and planting the vines close together—the highest-density plantings in Oregon (1,742 to 1,815 per acre, as opposed to 1,250 to 1,350 per acre for most vineyards)—which Saville feels also creates more structure and intensity of fruit in the wine. Because the vineyard is dry-farmed, Bishop Creek vines must reach deeper into the soil for water, making them more drought-resistant and less prone to splitting. Not to mention taste: All of these practices add up to higher-quality wines that show off this beautiful site.

Wines to Try: Bishop Creek Cellars has a tasting room called Urban Wine Works in Portland (at the address above), where you can taste its wines. Try the "Flight of the Week," so you can sample several of these delightful wines before you decide which one to go home with.

BRICK HOUSE VINEYARDS
DB · SS

18200 N.E. Lewis Rogers Lane · Newberg, OR 97132
(503) 538-5136 · www.brickhousewines.com

Owner Doug Tunnell calls his farm "a New World site dedicated to Old World wisdom." Biodynamic farming, he says, "has helped to enliven our soil and integrate our fields, blocks, microsites, gardens, landscapes into a single living and interdependent whole farm." He uses compost made from the remnants of the crush to fertilize the gardens and leaves from the oak grove feed the soil in the vineyard. "The result," Tunnell says, "is a vibrancy and life that we didn't enjoy in the years before we practiced biodynamics." He also sees a direct connection between his biodynamically farmed vineyard and the health of salmon streams. "The waters of the Willamette basin were once one of the world's greatest inland salmon spawning grounds," he writes. But farm runoff, says the US Geologic Survey, accounts for 60 percent of the pollutants in the Willamette River and its tributaries. Organic and biodynamic farming focus not only on keeping chemicals, herbicides, and pesticides out of streams but also mediating erosion with cover crops and other plantings. A longtime organic farmer, Tunnell has been a leader in the biodynamic movement in Oregon, assisting and guiding other winegrowers through the process of certification.

Wines to Try: One of Brick House's best wines is Les Dijonnais, made from 1994 plantings of Dijon clone Pinot Noir.

CAMERON WINERY
DRC · SS
8200 N.E. Worden Hill Road · Dundee, OR 97115
(503) 538-0336 · www.cameronwines.com

Winemaker John Paul's wines are made in the Burgundian tradition, which, to him, means that the grapes are grown without the use of irrigation, fermented with indigenous yeasts, and aged in small oak barrels—and of course French is spoken in the cellar. Paul sees his vineyards as a "closed loop" where all the animals, insects, flowers, stones, and vines work in concert to keep the farm running smoothly. He talks about every participant in the process as an essential partner: "Our goats provide the pulse of the farm, commenting on whatever is going on and sampling whatever plants we make available to them," he says. "Their principal occupation is blackberry removal and mowing down cover crop in the winter months."

Wines to Try: For a unique experience, try the Clos Electrique Chardonnay, made from grapes from rare French clones, fermented with native yeast (but finished with French yeast to ensure dryness), then aged in old oak barrels for two years. You have never tasted a Chardonnay like this.

CHEHALEM
OCSW · SS
Tasting Room: 106 S. Center Street · Newberg, OR 97132
(503) 538-4700
Winery: 31190 N.E. Veritas Lane · Newberg, OR 97132
(503) 537-5553 · www.chehalemwines.com

Chehalem's wines are grown in LIVE-certified, organically farmed vineyards, some of which are dry-farmed to reduce erosion and save water; the Corral Creek Vineyard is 60 percent dry-farmed and has not been irrigated for two years. Owners Harry Peterson-Nedry and Bill Stoller (also of Stoller Vineyards) are actively involved in the wine world in Oregon and at large, supporting the Oregon Wine Board and other organizations that promote growing the industry in a sustainable fashion. For instance, beyond practices of sustainable farming, this winery also sees packaging as a part of its responsibility to lower energy and waste. Working with Boise Cascade paper company, Chehalem developed an eight-sided corrugated cardboard box to eliminate Styrofoam inserts. The box carries a baker's dozen—or a winemaker's dozen—which lowers the number of boxes needed in a large shipment or allows for that much-loved sample bottle. In another win-win situation, Chehalem renovated a historic building in downtown Newberg, so people can taste its wines without having to drive so far (and use gas). The building includes a refurbished concrete floor and an eco-friendly

Chroma resin countertop, and displays the work of Portland glass artist Walter Gordinier.

Wines to Try: The INOX Chardonnay is a fresh, bright, minerally wine with no oak, and zesty aromatics, that goes wonderfully well with oysters and fresh seafood.

COOPER MOUNTAIN WINERY
CNC · CO · OTCO
9480 S.W. Grabhorn Road · Beaverton, OR 97007
(503) 649-0027 · www.coopermountainwine.com

Owners Robert and Corrine Gross have slowly brought their Cooper Mountain wines to the highest level of sustainable certifications, both in the vineyard and in the winery. They planted their first vines in 1978 and sold the grapes to wineries around Oregon. They established their winery in 1987, and now the vineyards have expanded to 123 acres, Demeter Certified Biodynamic since 1999. In the winery, they use soft cleaning agents and never use chlorine or iodine, which are prohibited by the National Organic Program.

Wines to Try: If you are looking for a completely sulfite-free wine, try Cooper Mountain Life Pinot Noir.

COWHORN
DB
1665 Eastside Road · Jacksonville, OR 97530
(541) 899-6876 · www.cowhornwine.com

Bill and Barbara Steele came to biodynamics in a different way than many. The couple were each working in New York City but often visited an uncle near Medford. They ultimately decided to find land and stay for good, starting an organic operation on an old 117-acre farm in the dry hills of southern Oregon, planting grapes in the stony soil of an old riverbed that extends beyond the current banks of the Applegate River. They had never farmed nor made wine, but Barbara connected with biodynamic farmers in Northern California and Oregon such as Doug Tunnell of Brick House Vineyards and consultant Alan York, who guided them through the process of creating a biodynamic farm. Now their aromatic, elegant Rhône-style Syrah, Grenache, and Viognier are winning many fans.

Wines to Try: Cowhorn Grenache is a gorgeous wine, with a purity of fresh red fruit—strawberry and raspberry flavors—with tannins Bill aptly describes as "raw silk," and a stony minerality that makes this wine a joy to savor.

CRISTOM
LIVE · OCSW · SS
6905 Spring Valley Road N.W. · Salem, OR 97304
(503) 375-3068 · www.cristomwines.com

For Cristom owner Paul Gerrie, vineyard manager Mark Letz, winemaker Steve Doerner, and their family of wine lovers, conservation in the winery is as important as a low-impact approach in the vineyard. The LIVE program also certifies for sustainable practices in the winery and, in Cristom's case, has encouraged the winemakers to use lighter, more eco-friendly glass and recycled materials, manage wastewater, and eliminate high-risk cleaning agents. Doerner has worked in wine regions around the world, including California, Chile, Italy, France, Germany, Australia, and New Zealand, and feels that Oregon is an incredible place to make wine for its diversity; Cristom's eight vineyards have been planted with not only Pinot and Chardonnay (staples in Oregon), but also with lovely Viognier and Syrah.

DOBBES FAMILY ESTATE
OCSW
240 S.E. 5th Street · Dundee, OR 97115
(503) 538-1141 · www.joedobbeswine.com

Over the past 25 years, Joe Dobbes has slowly grown his business into a 76,000-case-per-year operation, encompassing the affordable and delicious Wine by Joe and Jovino brands, as well as Dobbes Family Estate and the Joe Dobbes Collection. All this work has paid off in many ways, and in 2012, *Wine Business Monthly* named Wine by Joe the "Number One Hot Small Brand" in the nation. Sourcing from almost a dozen vineyards, the winemakers create simple, deliciously drinkable Pinot Noir and Pinot Gris under the Wine by Joe label, as well as premium, terroir-driven wines under the Dobbes Family label. The Larkins Estate Vineyard is LIVE certified; on the winery side, the custom winemaking facility was the first in the state of Oregon to earn this designation. Although the efforts of one winery, they say, may have a very small impact, "up close—in our tiny neck of the woods and in the hearts and minds of everyone connected to Dobbes Family Estate and Wine by Joe—it makes a world of difference."

DOMAINE DROUHIN
SS (estate wines)
6750 Breyman Orchards Road · Dayton, OR 97114
(503) 864-2700 · www.domainedrouhin.com

When Robert Drouhin, proprietor of Maison Joseph Drouhin in Burgundy, France, visited the Willamette Valley in 1961 and saw the soil and the climate, and then tasted Oregon wines throughout the 1970s, he felt that Oregon would be the next great place for Pinot Noir. Eventually, in 1987, his family purchased the property that would become Domaine Drouhin. Now his daughter Véronique is the winemaker, crafting feminine, elegant wines. Her brothers Frédéric, Philippe, and Laurent are involved in the business side in Burgundy and Oregon. Dedicated to growing their own rootstock, they have on-site nurseries and develop vines tailored to grow best in each particular block of the vineyards. Domaine Drouhin also features 500 solar panels, a 94.5-kilowatt ground-mounted system that, when installed, was the Oregon wine industry's largest.

DOMAINE DANIELLE LAURENT
DB
17100 N.E. Woodland Loop Road · Yamhill, Oregon 97148
(503) 662-4730 · www.solenaestate.com · www.thegrandcruestates.com

After making wine for many wineries in France and the States, including at WillaKenzie, Laurent Montalieu (whose last name, interestingly, means "mountain place") now has his own little place in the Dundee Hills. Most notably, he and his wife, Danielle Andrus Montalieu, have developed their 80-acre Domaine Danielle Laurent, a wedding present to each other, into a certified biodynamic vineyard. Laurent feels that the biodynamic practices of building soil and plant health through applying plant- and animal-waste-based compost-tea preparations have improved the health of their four-year-old vineyard's soil, and they are looking forward to creating dynamic Pinot Noir from these vineyards. At their Soléna winery—a name that combines the Spanish *solana* with their daughter's French name, Solene—the Montalieus currently produce Pinot Noir, Pinot Gris, Chardonnay, Cabernet Sauvignon, Merlot, Zinfandel, Syrah, and a late-harvest Riesling. They have another project at the winery called Grand Cru Estates, a membership-based winery with eco-friendly features like solar power and rainwater collection, where people can work with Laurent to make their personal barrel of Pinot Noir and experience life, and the art of winemaking, on this beautiful farm.

DOMAINE SERENE

6555 N.E. Hilltop Lane · Dayton, OR 97114
(503) 864-4600 · www.domaineserene.com
Proprietary program

Domaine Serene's Ken and Grace Evenstad believe that dry farming is essential to sustainable winegrowing practice. In Burgundy, irrigation is strictly forbidden, in order to ensure that the vines create a deep root system to help them survive in dry years and to create the highest-quality wine. "If one needs to divert rivers to irrigate vineyards," says Ken on the Domaine Serene website, "those vineyards are probably planted in the wrong place if they are meant to be sustainable." The Evanstads have created their own Sustainable Farming Practices Program that includes low crop yields and uses only natural products in the vineyard. On their 462-acre estate, 150 acres are planted in grapes, and more than half of the acreage is dedicated to wildlife habitat.

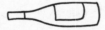

ELK COVE VINEYARDS

SS (estate wines)
27751 N.W. Olson Road · Gaston, OR 97119
(503) 985-7760 · www.elkcove.com

One of the oldest wineries in Oregon, Elk Cove creates many wines from its 220 acres of vineyards, all of which are farmed using various sustainable methods to varying degrees, from basic low-impact natural herbicides to complete organic standards. For instance, Windhill Vineyard has been organically farmed since 1999 but doesn't have organic certification. The other vineyards—La Bohème, Mount Richmond, Roosevelt, and Five Mountain—are farmed according to what are considered the needs of each.

Winemaker Adam Godlee Campbell, son of owners/growers Pat and Joe Campbell, came on board in 1995 to produce Elk Cove's excellent Pinot Noir and Pinot Gris. He grew up among the vines and feels that winemaking is a matter of "stewardship over intervention."

EVENING LAND VINEYARDS
DRC
572 Patterson Street N.W., Suite 170 · Salem, OR 97304
(503) 395-2520 · www.eveninglandvineyards.com
By appointment only · Biodynamic practices

When asked how biodynamic practices affect the wines at Evening Land, winemaker Isabelle Meunier said, in a *Portland Monthly* interview, "The principles of biodynamics are a philosophy—a belief in the quest for a memorable wine that can show a great sense of place. With regard to Chardonnay, I think that the best reward one can achieve is balance. I like to use a gentle and more natural approach, out of respect for the environment, the vineyard, and the fruit, with the goal to show elegance and let the wine speak for itself." For Evening Land, the minimal approach has paid off in excellent reviews and many new fans of these finessed wines. At the time of this writing, Evening Land Vineyards was working through the final stages of certification, after using the practices for several years.

Wines to Try: Tasting Evening Land Pinot Noir is a special experience. It is heady and floral, more aromatic than almost any wine, except Muscat, that I have ever tried. Violet and cherry blossom aromas entice, followed by a velvety smooth palate of cherry preserves, dried herbs, and wet stone. An enchanting wine.

EVESHAM WOOD
CO · DRC · SS
3795 Wallace Road N.W. · Salem, Oregon
(503) 371-8478 · www.eveshamwood.com
HADEN FIG
(503) 477-6960 · www.hadenfig.com

"At Evesham Wood," owners Russ and Mary Raney say, "small is beautiful." They have kept things simple at their 13-acre, certified organic vineyard since 1986. The vineyard, Le Puits Sec ("the dry well"), has been farmed organically since 2002, and the Raneys were charter members of the Deep Roots Coalition, an Oregon group that advocates natural methods and nonirrigated vineyards. In 2010, friends and Haden Fig winemakers Erin and Jordan Nuccio took over Evesham Wood, so Russ and Mary could obtain some much-needed retirement rest. Haden Fig is gaining fans for its delicious Pinot Noir and rosé wines. Winemaker Erin and his veterinarian wife, Jordan, make their wine at Evesham Wood and agree with the Raneys regarding the importance of organic, biodynamic, and other sustainable winegrowing and winemaking practices. Their label features the northern saw-whet owl, an important rodent predator in the vineyard, as a symbol of their commitment to sustainable agriculture.

JOHAN VINEYARDS
DB
4285 N. Pacific Highway (99W) · Rickreall, OR 97371
(866) 379-6029 · www.johanvineyards.com

One of the latest but most energetic additions to the Oregon wine scene is Johan Vineyards, named after proprietor Dag Johan Sundby, a young Norwegian who calls himself "the descendant of a long line of tillers of the soil" and who found a passion for Oregon Pinot Noir through an American family friend, Ray McCall. Johan has been farming biodynamically since 2005, and his winery is certified biodynamic, which means no additives may be added to the wines except minimal sulfites. Sundby likes to think of the job as managing the grapes through each phase of growth, from bloom to fruit set, to the "lag phase" (in which the grapes change from a vegetative mode to a fruiting mode and the seeds start to harden), through to verasion, or the ripening process. At each phase, the different biodynamic preparations, such as a tea made of fresh or fermented horsetail, are sprayed in small, homeopathic doses on the vineyard to stimulate growth or fend off fungus. These practices, according to biodynamics—and Sundby—create fruit that is healthy, pure tasting, and full of "life-force."

KING ESTATE WINERY
CO · OCSW
80854 Territorial Road · Eugene, OR 97405
(541) 942-9874 · www.kingestate.com

The largest organic vineyard in the state, King Estate comprises 1,033 certified organic acres. Among many other practices, the vineyards create 1,000 tons of compost a year from prunings, leaf clippings, pomace, and grapes that are dropped during preharvest pruning. No herbicides are used, and in addition, cover crops such as Austrian peas, crimson clover, wheat, oats, and flowering perennials are grown from organic seed in the gardens, to attract beneficial insects and create biodiversity and erosion control. The most effective pest control, however, is the rehabilitated barn owls, screech owls, and American kestrels living in the eight raptor boxes installed around the property by the Cascades Raptor Center in 2009. The inspiration came from a seminar the CRC conducted the year before that attracted 200 people and made it obvious that King Estate, with its biodiversity and large acreage, was the perfect place for raptors to thrive and do their part in the making of great wine.

LEFT COAST CELLARS
CNC
4225 N. Pacific Highway (99W) · Rickreall, OR 97371
(503) 831-4916 · www.leftcoastcellars.com

Left Coast Cellars is in Rickreall, central Oregon and, as they say, directly on the 45th parallel. The 306-acre farm has other crops besides grapes (such as European truffles) and includes a 4-acre site of hazelnut trees, shrub roses, and holly oaks. A grove of olive trees and an organic vegetable garden help stock the Tasting Room Café. This beautiful site with lakes, streams, and fields is also home to one of the last stands of original old-growth white oaks. Left Coast is currently working on becoming LIVE certified.

LEMELSON VINEYARDS
CNC · CO
12020 N.E. Stag Hollow Road · Carlton, Oregon 97111
(503) 852-6619 · www.lemelsonvineyards.com

Lemelson is using the sun to grow more than just grapes. In November 2007, it installed a 50-kilowatt solar electric system at the winery, providing up to 40 percent of the power needs of its main building on an annual basis. It is involved in the Carbon Neutral Challenge and, in the winery, has used sustainably grown and produced lumber from Collins Lumber, an Oregon-based family-owned timber company. Other wood, such as oak flooring, came from trees on the property. Lemelson Vineyards has been certified organic since 2004.

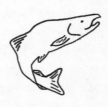

• •

NORA'S TABLE: LOCAVORE WINES

The quaint town of Hood River, Oregon, in the Columbia Gorge, is perfectly positioned for wine touring. The Columbia Gorge AVA, established in 2004, is getting to be better known for its varied and excellent wines and fascinating geography and geology. The Columbia Gorge Winegrowers Association's tagline sums it up well: "A world of wine in 40 miles!" It adds "just one gorgeous hour from Portland." Vines grow atop sheer 600-foot cliffs on either side of the massive river, basking in the long, hot days. At night, the river helps to cool down the grapes and retain acidity and fresh, pure flavors. About 30 vineyards and about 30 wineries call the Gorge AVA home.

At one Hood River restaurant, Nora's Table, founder and chef Kathy Watson has taken the "locavore" movement into the wine cellar by creating a unique "Gorge only" wine list. "There is such an excellent selection of wines available from the wineries in the Columbia River Gorge," Watson says, "there's no sustainable reason to buy imports from South America, Australia, or even California." The delightfully varied list includes Old Vine Zinfandel from The Pines 1852 Winery, Marchesi Vineyards' Sangiovese, the biodynamic Dominio IV's Technicolor Bat red blend, all from the Oregon side, and Syncline Viognier, Domaine Pouillon's Black Dot red blend, and Memaloose Cabernet Franc from the Washington side.

Watson also buys most, if not all, of her produce, fish, and meat from as close as possible. She sees this as the way to create a local "Columbia Gorge cuisine" by using what is grown locally and taking risks such as making a salad out of strawberries and thinly sliced radishes because they are both in their prime at the same time. "This is how restaurants and farmers are creating a Gorge cuisine," Watson writes in a great essay on her blog called "The Thrill of the Mystery Box: How Proximity and Inspiration Create Cuisine." "Chefs are more willing to take risks with food and in fact, our diners expect it of us. They want to see us try new things, and perhaps inspire them to cut thin rounds of radishes and thin rounds of strawberries and toss them together."

Nora's Table is inspirational in many ways beyond its delicious Gorge cuisine. It has created a business that is based in community and has built bridges between farmers, winegrowers, winemakers, home cooks, and those of us who want to support the people whose passion it is to bring us such delicious locally—and sustainably—grown food and wine.

· ·

LUMOS WINE COMPANY
FA · SS (Temperance Hill, Wren Vineyards)
24000 Cardwell Hill Drive · Philomath, OR 97370
(541) 929-6257 · www.lumoswine.com

Dai Crisp has earned the title *vigneron*, French for winegrower. He grows all the grapes that go into his wines, including elegant Pinot Noirs and refreshing Pinot Gris, using only natural fertilizers and no chemical herbicides or systemic fungicides. His three vineyards—Temperance Hill, Logsdon Ridge, and Wren—contain some of the oldest vines in Oregon, with plantings back to 1980. He and his "Grand Crew," which includes his wife, P. K. McCoy, and their three children, Dominique, Boone, and Katie, plus a core team of vineyard tenders, grow pampered grapes according to Oregon Tilth organic standards.

Wines to Try: Temperance Vineyard produces delicate and interesting Pinot Noir wines, with mineral and floral, bright-cherry, and earth aromas. The Pinot Noir Rosé is a refreshing and delightful pairing with cold chicken or spot-prawn salad.

MAHONIA VINEYARDS
CNC · LIVE · SS
4985 Battle Creek Road S.E. · Salem, OR 97302
(503) 585-8789 · www.mahoniavineyard.com

John Miller, owner of Mahonia Vineyards (named after the Oregon state flower, *Mahonia aquifolium*, or Oregon grape), was one of the early adopters of contemporary—and traditional—sustainable farming practices in Oregon. He planted an 11-acre farm in 1985, farming without pesticides or herbicides and selling the fruit to top Oregon Pinot Noir producers, including Evesham Wood, which used it in a vineyard-designated wine. Miller's focus on organics in the vineyard and energy savings in the winery has led him to install solar panels and use biodeisel to power winery vehicles. Winemaker Chris Berg (from Roots Winery and Vineyard) now crafts Mahonia Vineyard fruit into small lots of Pinot Noir, Pinot Gris, and Chardonnay from grapes that have been attracting winemakers, and now wine lovers, for years.

MAYSARA WINERY / MOMTAZI VINEYARD
DB

15765 S.W. Muddy Valley Road · McMinnville, OR 97128
(503) 843-1234 · www.maysara.com

It might seem difficult to apply biodynamic methods to a huge 540-acre farm, but according to Moe Momtazi, "The hardest part is gaining the knowledge and understanding of biodynamics. When you reach this, it is easy to implement the practices throughout the entire farm. It is important to not pick and choose the pieces you want to follow, but to practice this process in its entirety." Momtazi feels as if it has paid off in much-improved soil, more evenly and fully ripened fruit, and a sense that he is farming the land in a responsible way and letting it find its own balance. In the winery, he lets both primary and secondary (malolactic) fermentation begin on their own, rather than adding anything such as yeast or bacteria to begin these processes. As a result, the wines are a purer reflection of the fruit and the terroir of the vineyard, without outside influences.

MONTINORE ESTATE
DB · OCSW
3663 S.W. Dilley Road · Forest Grove, OR 97116
(503) 359-5012 ext. 3 · www.montinore.com

According to Demeter International, one thing that sets apart certified-biodynamic farms is "whole farm certification" rather than just certifying a particular crop area. Montinore's proprietor, Rudy Marchesi, has owned his 230-acre vineyard since 2001, and when he took it over, the soil had been depleted of organic matter and nutrients. He started working on reviving the soil and vines and has been certified biodynamic since 2008. "The soils used to be heavily compacted, meaning water would run right off," he says. "Within a year after we started using biodynamic preparations here, you could sink a shovel into the ground without any effort at all. The difference was amazing." He feels the wines have benefited, too, with fresher, brighter flavors and aromas. Montinore is also a member of the Oregon Certified Sustainable Wine program, which incorporates LIVE and Salmon-Safe certifications. Of the 230 acres, 123 are planted in Pinot Noir, Pinot Gris, Riesling, Müller-Thurgau, and Gewürztraminer; these cool-climate grapes thrive in the shadow of Oregon's coastal mountain range and make delightfully refreshing and elegant wines.

SOKOL BLOSSER
CNC · LEED · OCSW · SS (estate wines)
5000 N.E. Sokol Blosser Lane · Dayton, OR 97114
(503) 864-2282 · www.sokolblosser.com

Sustainability is not just for the vineyard. In 2002, Sokol Blosser's underground barrel rooms made this the first US winery to receive LEED certification. One hundred percent of the winery and office energy comes from renewable sources such as solar and wind. In its 2011 annual sustainability report, Sokol Blosser reported that through the PGE Clean Wine Program it offset 62,656 pounds of CO_2, which equates roughly to 69,656 miles not driven or 3,765 trees planted. Another interesting program is the Conservation Reserve Enhancement Program (CREP), a "voluntary land retirement program that helps agricultural producers protect environmentally sensitive land, decrease erosion, restore wildlife habitat, and safeguard ground and surface water." Sokol Blosser sets six acres of land aside, planting about 1,000 trees and eradicating invasive species such as English ivy, non-native blackberries, and poison oak. This is all in support of organic and some biodynamic winegrowing, producing complex and delicious wines.

SOTER VINEYARDS
CNC · OCSW · SS
10880 N.E. Mineral Springs Road · Carlton, OR 97111
(503) 852-6944 · www.sotervineyards.com

Tony Soter was a consulting winemaker in Napa for years, working with great wineries such as Araujo, Niebaum-Coppola, Shafer, Spottswoode, Viader, and Dalle Valle. He finally struck out on his own, purchasing vineyards in Oregon's Willamette Valley and setting out to make world-class wine with low environmental impact. He was on the steering committee for the Carbon Neutral Challenge, and his vineyard is free of pesticides and herbicides, hoping to let the fruit shine in the wine. Soter is also involved in the Planet Oregon Wine project, a separate label that donates $1 per bottle of sustainably produced Planet Oregon Pinot Noir to the Oregon Environmental Council. In 2011 it donated $5,400, with hopes for more in the coming years. Tony's wife and partner, Michelle Soter, feels this program brings together many of their ideals: "It is a continuing goal to foster responsible agricultural practices and the awareness of healthy choices in food and wine consumption."

SALUD! SUSTAINING OREGON'S VINEYARD WORKERS

"Vineyard workers are absolutely the base of our whole industry," says Ronni Lacroute of WillaKenzie Estate in the Willamette Valley. Pruning, thinning, and harvesting a vineyard is backbreaking work done by actual people, often seasonal workers who are paid little. A particular hazard is chemicals: For years, chemical fertilizers, herbicides, and pesticides were seen as easy ways to manage crops and create profit, but grapes aren't the only things affected by these chemicals—they take their toll on people, too. (Whether in small family wineries or large corporations, often the decision to use fewer chemical inputs is made in order to keep workers healthier.)

Most of these seasonal workers, many of whom travel from harvest to harvest, have no medical insurance or access to medical care and can suffer from work-related injuries and illnesses. The idea of the "triple bottom line," or "people, planet, and profit," is used to describe the balance needed for creating an environmentally, socially, and economically sustainable business, but the wine industry, like other agricultural industries, continues to have its issues in each of these areas. Still, with immigration laws and industry growth generating worker shortages all along the West Coast, many wineries are doing more to keep their workers and to keep their workers happy and healthy.

Oregon nonprofit Salud! is trying to address these issues. Dedicated to "providing access to healthcare services for Oregon's seasonal vineyard workers and their families," Salud! is the most extensive program of its kind, a partnership between Tuality Healthcare Foundation and 40 percent of the wineries in Oregon. Vineyard workers "give us fair work, honesty, loyalty, everything," says Nancy Ponzi of Ponzi Winery in Dundee, Oregon, "and we have an obligation to give it back to them." Funded by the annual Pinot Noir auction and sales of specially crafted blends made exclusively for that auction, Salud! raised $670,000 in its 2010 auction and and has raised more than $9 million since its beginning in 1991.

In 2011 alone, Salud! provided services to more than 3,600 workers and their families, with a total of more than 7,000 medical visits, including dental procedures, flu and tetanus vaccinations, vision exams, X-rays, first-aid classes, and major medical services such as surgery and hospitalizations. Thanks to collaborations with healthcare organizations, Salud! is able to deliver $3 in value for every $1 spent. It is truly a model of the "people" side of sustainability for the whole industry. As Amy Wesselman of Westrey Vineyards says, "If wine is made in the vineyard, then we have to take care of the people who make it in the vineyard."

STOLLER VINEYARDS
CNC · OCSW
6161 N.E. McDougall Road · Dayton, OR 97114
(503) 864-3404 · www.stollervineyards.com

Bill Stoller's father and uncle ran a turkey farm on the 373-acre property that is now Stoller Vineyards, and they used to complain that their soil was not as rich as that of surrounding farms, that there were too many rocks, and the hills were too steep. By the time Stoller grew up, he figured out that this land in the Dundee Hills of the Willamette Valley could make a prime vineyard site. In fact, those "problems" were all pluses for wine grapes—that and the lifetime supply of natural fertilizer the turkeys had worked into the soil. Stoller bought the land from a cousin in 1993 and in 1995 planted his first Chardonnay grapes. In 2006, Stoller built the first LEED Gold–certified winery in the United States, incorporating a gravity-flow winemaking system so the grapes and juice don't have to be pumped to reach their tanks, as well as energy-efficient heating and cooling and wastewater reclamation. Stoller Pinot Noirs are full of bright-red fruit flavors, with complex mineral, mushroom, and tobacco notes.

VAN DUZER VINEYARDS
LIVE · SS
11975 Smithfield Road · Dallas, OR 97338
(800) 884-1927 · www.vanduzer.com

In 1998, Van Duzer Vineyards started adopting sustainable winegrowing practices in its 82-acre vineyard; among other results, it has cut water usage by 30 percent. In 2006 they built a new 20,000-case winery, employing many eco-friendly elements. The cellar is half buried in the hillside and maintains constant temperatures year-round, minimizing energy use. There's also a highly reflective roof to keep heat out, and chemical-free winery production water is used to irrigate the vines. The owners, Carl and Marilynn Thoma, looked a long while for this site, and they feel it is a perfect place for great Pinot Noir wines. The wines are always interesting, complex, and balanced, with delicate, pure fruit.

Wines to Try: Van Duzer's beautiful labels reflect the ephemeral, elegant quality of its wines. With the 2010 vintage, the winery focused on super-gentle handling of the fruit, meant to capture Pinot Noir's delicate aromas. It succeeded, with captivating smoky spice, black tea, and red fruit aromas.

. . . .

JIMI BROOKS: A LEGACY OF EXPERIMENTATION AND INSPIRATION

Jimi Brooks is a legend in the young history of Oregon wine. By the time of his tragic death at age 38, from a heart aneurism during the 2004 harvest, he had already affected so many lives in the close-knit Oregon wine business that his loss was felt across the state and throughout the industry. Wine writer Katherine Cole called him, "one of those wickedly funny, effortlessly likable people who could convince just about anyone to try just about anything."

After working in the Beaujolais region of France and learning about vineyard practices there, Brooks returned to Oregon in 1996 and became assistant winemaker for WillaKenzie Estate. He encouraged his friends winemaker Laurent Montalieu (now of Soléna Winery) and Jay Somers of J. Christopher Winery to experiment and learn more about biodynamics. In 1998, he started his own label, Brooks. In 2000, he went on to become vineyard manager and winemaker for Moe Momtazi of Momtazi Vineyards/Maysara Winery, and he was instrumental in working toward their Demeter certification in 2007.

Around the year 2000, Brooks worked with 5 acres of grapes and experimented with biodynamic practices at Eola Hills. He found that this approach produced better, riper fruit, healthier plants, and overall production of better and more consistent quality. Brooks said, "I believe that farming in this way, by keeping the earth alive and the ecosystem intact, is the only way to really achieve that concept of 'terroir.' While I respect the individuality of each piece of land and the sense of place, I believe one can achieve the greatest depth, flavors, and balance in a wine only by blending." Under the Brooks label, he made lovely, elegant wines from Pinot Noir and Riesling, first working with grapes he purchased from organic vineyards.

Many feel that if it weren't for Brooks's initial enthusiasm about the potential for growing great grapes using biodynamic methods that see the farm as a self-sustaining whole, using special preparations made from herbs and other plants grown right on the farm, and banning the use of all pesticides and herbicides, the history of sustainability in Oregon might have been different. His sister, Janie Brooks Heuck, and winemaker Chris Williams have continued Brooks winery and, since 2009, also own Eola Hills Vineyard, working it with biodynamic practices (not certified at the time of this writing, but it may become so), trying to honor a brother and friend for his vision and passion for the community he loved and that loved him.

- -

VIDON VINEYARD
LIVE · SS
17425 N.E. Hillside Drive · Newberg, OR 97132
(503) 538-4092 · www.vidonvineyard.com

Don and Vicky Hagge had a dream to make wine in Oregon as good as that which they had tasted in Burgundy. Their small 20-acre vineyard in the Chehalem Mountains produces just 1,300 cases per year, but they are still committed to keeping everything as pure as possible. They hand-pick their grapes and allow spontaneous fermentation to take place rather than adding commercial yeast to the fruit. Vidon is also LIVE certified, as well as Salmon-Safe. This small winery is also part of the Carbon Neutral Challenge, with efficient heating and cooling and solar panel energy.

WILLAMETTE VALLEY VINEYARDS
CO · LIVE · OCSW · SS (Elton, Hannah, Tualatin, and Willamette Valley estate vineyards)
8800 Enchanted Way S.E. · Turner, OR 97392
(503) 588-9463 · www.wvv.com

The folks at Willamette Valley Vineyards have been hard at work making their winery and vineyards more sustainable. For instance, besides growing grapes organically in the estate vineyard and gaining LIVE and Salmon-Safe certification for much of their vineyards, they also work with the Cascade Raptor Center to encourage owls and other raptors to lower gopher and other rodent populations without rodenticides. Led by founder Jim Bernau, the efforts don't stop there: WWV is also focused on recycling, with a 10-cent recycling refund for each bottle and $1 for returned shippers. It has also partnered with Amorim Cork America, the Oregon community-minded nonprofit SOLV (Stop Oregon Litter and Vandalism), and manufacturer Yemm and Hart to start a nationwide cork recycling program. Its cork is the first (and, at the time of this writing, the only) in the world to be certified through Rainforest Alliance Forest Stewardship Council (FSC) standards. Beyond drinking these delicious wines, the public can be involved in WWV's sustainability programs by sharing its ideas with the winery's Environmental Impact Committee, which meets quarterly to find new ways to lower its impact on the land.

WINDERLEA VINEYARD AND WINERY
CNC · LIVE · SS
8905 N.E. Worden Hill Road · Dundee, OR 97115
(503) 554-5900 · www.winderlea.com

Although not (as of the time of this writing) Demeter Certified Biody-namic, Winderlea is a great example of a newer winery in continual tran-sition toward sustainability. It brought on famed French biodynamic con-sultant Philippe Armenier in 2009 to advise on converting its vineyards to this "whole-farm approach that combines intense natural practices commonly found in organic farming along with the addition of unique preparations intended to stimulate plant and biological life as well as to bring the farm into balance with the natural rhythms of the earth, the sun, the moon, and the other planets." Along with owners Bill Sweat and Donna Morris, winemaker Robert Brittan (who also has his own vine-yards and winery) is focusing on creating premium Pinot Noir and Char-donnay wines that reflect this special place.

OTHER OREGON WINERIES WITH GREEN CONSIDERATIONS

ANTICA TERRA
979 S.W. Alder Street
Dundee, OR 97115
(503) 244-1748
www.anticaterra.com
Some biodynamic practices

ARBORBROOK VINEYARDS
17770 N.E. Calkins Lane
Newberg, OR 97132
(503) 538-0959
www.arborbrookwines.com
SS

BEAUX FRÈRES
15155 N.E. North Valley Road
Newberg, OR 97132
(503) 537-1137
www.beauxfreres.com
DRC

BELLE PENTE
12470 N.E. Rowland Road
Carlton, OR 97111
(503) 852-9500
www.bellepente.com
DRC
Some biodynamic practices

BRITTAN VINEYARDS
18580 Muddy Valley Road
McMinnville, Oregon 97128
(503) 989-2507
www.brittanvineyards.com

BROOKS
9360 S.E. Eola Hills Road
Amity, OR 97101
(503) 435-1278
www.brookswine.com
Biodynamic practices

CARDWELL HILL CELLARS
24241 Cardwell Hill Drive
Philomath, OR 97370
(541) 929-9463
www.cardwellhillwine.com
LIVE

CARLTON CELLARS
130 W. Monroe Street
Carlton, OR 97111
(503) 852-7888
www.carletoncellars.com

COELHO WINERY
111 5th Street
Amity, OR 97101
(503) 835-9305
www.coelhowinery.com
SS

DOMINIO IV
845 N.E. 5th Street
McMinnville OR 97128
(503) 474-8636
www.dominiowines.com
DB

EOLA HILLS
501 S. Pacific Highway W.
Rickreall, OR 97371
(503) 623-2405
www.eolahillswinery.com
SS

THE EYRIE VINEYARDS
935 N.E. 10th Avenue
McMinnville, OR 97128
(503) 472-6315
www.eyrievineyards.com
DRC

THE FOUR GRACES
9605 N.E. Fox Farm Road
Dundee, Oregon 97115
(800) 245-2950
www.thefourgraces.com
LIVE

ILLAHE VINEYARDS
3275 Ballard Road
Dallas, OR 97338
(503) 831-1248
www.illahevineyards.com
DRC · LIVE · SS

KRAMER VINEYARDS
26830 N.W. Olson Road
Gaston, OR 97119
(503) 662-4545
www.kramervineyards.com
LIVE · SS

LANGE ESTATE WINERY
18380 N.E. Buena Vista Drive
Dundee, OR 97115
(503) 538-6476
www.langewinery.com
LIVE · SS

OWEN ROE
8400 Champoeg Road N.E.
Saint Paul, OR 97137
(503) 678-6514
www.owenroe.com
SS (Cabernet, Riesling, Merlot)

PANTHER CREEK CELLARS
455 N.E. Irvine Street
McMinnville, OR 97128
(503) 472-8080
www.panthercreekcellars.com
OCSW · SS (Elton Vineyard only)

PATTON VALLEY VINEYARD
9449 S.W. Old Highway 47
Gaston, OR 97119
(503) 985-3445
www.pattonvalley.com
OCSW

PENNER-ASH WINE CELLARS
15771 N.E. Ribbon Ridge Road
Newberg, OR 97132
(503) 554-5545
www.pennerash.com
OCSW

PONZI VINEYARDS
14665 S.W. Winery Lane
Beaverton, OR 97007
(503) 628-1227
www.ponziwines.com
OCSW

REX HILL (see A to Z Wineworks)
30835 N. Highway 99W
Newberg, OR 97132
(503) 538-0666
www.rexhill.com
DB · OCSW

SINEANN
28005 N.E. Bell Road
Newberg, OR 97132
(503) 341-2698
www.sineann.com
SS (Resonance Vineyard)

SPINDRIFT CELLARS
810 Applegate Street
Philomath, OR 97370
(541) 929-6555
www.spindriftcellars.com
SS

TERRITORIAL VINEYARDS & WINE COMPANY
907 W. 3rd Avenue
Eugene, OR 97402
(541) 684-9463
www.territorialvineyards.com
SS

THREE ANGELS VINEYARD/ ANGEL VINE WINE
Available for tasting at:
Carlton Cellars
130 W. Monroe Street
Carlton, OR 97111
(503) 852-7888
www.angelvine.net
OCSW

TORII MOR WINERY
18323 N.E. Fairview Drive
Dundee, OR 97115
(503) 554-0105
www.toriimorwinery.com
OCSW

TRIUM WINERY
7112 Rapp Lane
Talent, OR 97540
(541) 535-4015
www.triumwines.com
SS

TROON VINEYARD
1475 Kubli Road
Grants Pass, OR 97527
(541) 846-9900
www.troonvineyard.com
SS

TYEE WINE CELLARS
26335 Greenberry Road
Corvallis, OR 97333
(541) 753-8754
www.tyeewine.com

VISTA HILLS VINEYARD & WINERY
6475 N.E. Hilltop Lane
Dayton, OR 97114
(503) 864-3200
www.vistahillsvineyard.com
LIVE · SS

WATERMILL WINERY
235 E. Broadway Avenue
Milton-Freewater, OR 97862
(541) 938-5575
www.watermillwinery.com
LIVE · SS (estate wines)

WESTREY WINE COMPANY
1065 N.E. Alpine Avenue
McMinnville, OR 97128
(503) 434-6357
www.westrey.com
DB (Momtazi Vineyard) · DRC ·
LIVE (Oracle Vineyard, Justice
Vineyard)

WILLAKENZIE ESTATE
19143 N.E. Laughlin Road
Yamhill, OR 97148
(503) 662-3280
www.willakenzie.com
OCSW

WINTER'S HILL VINEYARD
6451 N.E. Hilltop Lane
Dayton, OR 97114
(503) 864-4538
www.wintershillwine.com
SS

WITNESS TREE VINEYARD
7111 Spring Valley Road N.W.
Salem, OR 97304
(503) 585-7874
www.witnesstreevineyard.com
SS

**WOOLDRIDGE CREEK
VINEYARD & WINERY**
818 Slagle Creek Road
Grants Pass, OR 97527
(541) 846-6364
www.wcwinery.com
OCSW

YOUNGBERG HILL
10660 S.W. Youngberg Hill Road
McMinnville, OR 97128
(503) 472-2727
www.youngberghill.com
LIVE · SS
Biodynamic practices

ZERBA CELLARS
85530 Highway 11
Milton-Freewater, OR 97862
(541) 938-WINE
Dundee Tasting Room:
810 Highway 99W
Dundee, OR 97115
(503) 537-WINE
Woodinville Tasting Room:
14525 148th Avenue N.E.
Woodinville, WA 98072
(425) 806-2749
www.zerbacellars.com
LIVE · SS (estate wines) · VINEA

WASHINGTON WINERIES

Poor soil is great for grapes, right? This is what we always hear, that it's good to "stress" the vines, to make them reach deep for water and keep their leaf production (their "vigor") low. So the recent trend in talk about "soil building" seems like a shift in thinking, especially in Washington, where the volcanic, mineral-rich soil is often poor in nutrients, which often makes it necessary to amend the soil with organic matter and fertilizers. Luckily, Washington growers have been blessed with a dry, hot climate with low pest, weed, and disease pressure, so many Washington growers use minimal herbicides and pesticides.

Until recently, "sustainability" wasn't a commonly used word in Washington wineries' educational and marketing vocabularies. Many of the practices have been used by some all along—there are several growers and wineries that have been organic since the 1980s, Powers and Snoqualmie to name a couple. But it didn't seem to be a priority in the Washington industry at large until the past few years. This state, with its history of conventional apple and wheat farming emerging from the post–World War II penchant for chemical inputs, wasn't on the leading edge of chemical-free grape growing.

Following Oregon and California's lead, Washington now has 1,000 certified Salmon-Safe acres in Walla Walla and more than triple that throughout the state. The Washington Association of Grape Growers (WWAG) started VineWise in 2003, originally as a risk management organization to deal with issues surrounding insurance, contracts, human resources, business plans, marketing plans, water management, soil surface, and soil management. Since then, however, after creating a series of checklists for growers on those subjects, VineWise has expanded to address issues of sustainability in the vineyard and in the business realm.

Currently, Snoqualmie Winery winemaker Joy Anderson is overseeing the development of Winerywise, a program for sustainability in the winery as well. It embraces the implementation of third-party LIVE certification, and slowly, more and more vineyards and wineries are joining in the process of self-evaluation and improving viniculture processes. Winegrowers evaluate pressures from disease, weeds, and pests such as the Western grape leafhopper, Virginia creeper leafhopper, grape mealybug, cutworms, mites, and thrips, to determine how they can lower their use of pesticides by encouraging beneficial insects and using less harmful products.

It is interesting to note that of the two dozen or so vineyards and wineries that are certified biodynamic in the United States, four are in Washington: Aecetia Vineyard (Naches Heights Winery), Hedges Estate Vineyard, Wallula Gap (Pacific Rim Winery), and Wilridge Vineyard (Wilridge Winery). Christophe Baron of Cayuse Vineyards was the area's pioneer (his vineyards are over the border in the Oregon section of the Walla Walla Valley, but the winery is bonded in Washington), and although he has chosen to no longer be certified, he is still one of the most passionate voices for biodynamics and practices it fully in his vineyard and farm.

ABEJA
SS · VINEA
2014 Mill Creek Road · Walla Walla, WA 99362
(509) 526-7400 · www.abeja.net

Named after the Spanish word for "bee," Abeja has been busy producing gorgeous wines since 2002. Winemaker John Abbott has a particular gift for creating elegant wines with impressive balance and finesse. He started by buying fruit but ultimately planted the 17-acre Heather Hill estate vineyard with strict attention to sustainability, using no chemical fertilizers herbicides or pesticides in the vineyard, and planting for beneficial insects to help control the unwelcome ones. Abeja released its first vineyard-designated wine in 2011, a 100 percent Cabernet Sauvignon. It also sources fruit from some of the Columbia Valley's best vineyards; Abbott's judicious used of oak, and insistence on balancing acidity and tannins, makes these wines a great example of the elegance Washington fruit can attain. But Abeja is more than just a winery. Owners Ken and Ginger Harrison bought the nearby Mill Creek Inn bed-and-breakfast, northwest of Walla Walla, in 2000 and continued the restoration of several farmhouses and a huge barn on the century-old property. Abbott and his partner Molly Galt, who runs the inn, joined the Harrisons as partners in 2002. The restoration continued, with a focus on reclaimed wood and salvaged materials to retain the farmstead feel, while giving the property a boutique-like quality beyond its original glory. Abeja's Heather Hill estate vineyard was one of the earliest Vinea-certified vineyards, and it takes its stewardship of this historic property and watershed seriously.

Wines to Try: The estate-grown Viognier is full of lush stone fruit but with a backbone of fresh acidity that can be lacking in Washington Viognier. The Syrah is another estate wine, grown right on the winery grounds, nestled at 1,310 feet in elevation in the foothills of the Blue Mountains. This cooler site helps the Syrah avoid flabbiness, by gaining acidity and ripening slowly.

ÀMAURICE CELLARS
SS
178 Vineyard Lane · Walla Walla, WA 99362
(509) 522-5444 · www.àMaurice.com

Just up the country road from Abeja, àMaurice Cellars has been a leader in sustainable practices in Walla Walla. The Schafer family—Tom and

Kathleen, and their children Anna, Nicholas, and Stephanie—established their winery in 2004. For two years before planting their 13.5-acre vineyard of Viognier, Syrah, Malbec, and Cabernet Sauvignon, they "just grew dirt" according to Anna, observing the wind from the Blue Mountains and the soil quality and considering "how to best steward the vines to produce their best." Working with vineyard manager Ken Hart and soil consultant Rick Trumbull, they continue to build the soil and health of their vineyard, and engage in their "ongoing love affair with its dirt." Led by Anna's enthusiasm for winemaking and sustainable farming, àMaurice was a charter member of Vinea: The Winegrowers' Sustainable Trust and embraced the Salmon-Safe movement early on. For several winters, Anna has worked in Mendoza, Argentina, with winemaker Paul Hobbs's Viña Cobos winery, speeding her winemaking education and gaining kudos along the way. "We are dedicated to sustainable farming and stewardship of the land," says Anna. "We want to make sure that in a hundred years, this is still here."

Wines to Try: For sustainable options, try the estate-grown wines, especially the Malbec, with its lush blueberry and blackberry fruit, smoke, and earthy minerality, which gained Steven Tanzer's blessing as "the best Malbec in the United States." The small-production, estate-grown Sparrow Viognier is all lush peach, sweet spice, and flowers.

AMAVI CELLARS
LIVE · SS
3796 Peppers Bridge Road · Walla Walla, WA 99362
(509) 525-3541 · www.amavicellars.com

Amavi is a second-generation winery, you might say. Norm McKibben and Ray Goff's Pepper Bridge Winery, which makes Cabernet and Merlot varietal wines and blends, amounts to Amavi's father: McKibben's and Goff's children, Eric and Shane McKibben and Travis Goff, are partners with Pepper Bridge winemaker Jean-François Pellet and draw from the same estate vineyards: Pepper Bridge, Seven Hills, Les Collines, and Goff. The wines are as good as Pepper Bridge's but focus more on Syrah, with some Sémillon, late-harvest Sémillon, and rosé available. Surprisingly, for a winery in Washington to make 100 percent estate, sustainably grown wines is not too common, and Pepper Bridge and Amavi are sister labels that accomplish that goal admirably. Pellet's winemaking style is to let the fruit sing, and his wines are very balanced, with bright acidity and not too much oak or alcohol. These wines are also less pricey than Pepper Bridge's, presenting a great opportunity to experience Pellet's artistic palette for less.

BADGER MOUNTAIN VINEYARD/POWERS WINERY
CO (Badger Mountain Vineyard)
1106 N. Jurupa Street · Kennewick, WA 99338
(800) 643-WINE · www.badgermountainvineyard.com

When Bill Powers planted his 80-acre vineyard with his son Greg in 1982, he was ahead of his time; in 1990, Badger Mountain Vineyard became the first certified organic vineyard in Washington State. Since then, Badger Mountain wines slowly have been finding a following, both in the organic wine aisle and beyond. In the vineyard right outside the door Badger Mountain uses sustainable practices such as composting, using compost teas, burning weeds, using an in-row cultivator instead of applying herbicides, using pest fans to blow bugs off plants instead of using pesticides, introducing beneficial insects, planting cover crops, and spreading grape pomace and skins back into the vineyard. Packaging is also a big part of the plan; it introduced some of the first box wines in the country for the Pure White and Pure Red organic wines. Winemaker Jose Mendoza and Director of Winemaking Greg Powers have an NSA (No Sulfites Added) series for people who may be sensitive to sulfites. The Powerses also created another label, Powers, which focuses on producing premium wines, such as Champoux Vineyard Chardonnay, from top Washington vineyards, but don't have an overt "sustainability" message.

CHRISTOPHE HEDGES: REVOLUTIONARY WINE SON

Christophe Hedges is a dynamo of the wine world. The son of Hedges Family Estate owners Tom and Anne-Marie Hedges, he has been a bull rider and a wine steward at Costco (jobs that need similar skills) and has a business degree and a minor in theater arts. It all makes sense, since Christophe has taken his family's business from a traditional, quality-focused family winery to one that is making waves in the wine world.

Hedges Family Estate is the first Washington winery to have a certified-biodynamic vineyard (Cayuse Vineyard was the first in the region; the vineyard is over the border in Oregon and farms biodynamically). Although it makes 90 percent of its wines from noncertified vineyards, it is moving in a sustainable direction. As for Christophe, he is shaking up the wine-scene hierarchy with his Score Revolution project, which aims at "saving place of origin with elegance." The revolution is an anti-wine-scoring campaign, against the *Wine Spectators* and Robert Parkers of the world, who, according to Hedges, have oversimplified wine for the consumer and created an atmosphere in which winemakers create wines to suit a particular critic's palate, i.e., specifically the "Parkerization" of wine, by which big, fruity, dark wines are given higher scores than lighter, more delicately aromatic ones. In the Score Revolution Manifesto (which you can sign and discuss at www.scorevolution.com), Hedges writes:

> The 100 point rating system is a clumsy and useless tool
> for examining wine. If wine is, as we believe, a subjective,
> subtle, and experiential thing, then by nature it is unquanti-
> fiable. Wine scores are merely a static symbol, an absolute

*definition based on a singular contact with a wine, and thus
completely ineffective when applied to a dynamic, evolving,
and multifaceted produce.*

How does this relate to sustainability? Hedges believes that over-manipulation in the vineyard and winery replaces the grape's natural expression with artificial flavors and aromas meant to please a certain market. Indeed, much of the wine world works this way. Thus, rejecting the status quo of wine scores is a step toward more "natural" winemaking, so that the complex, "infinitely variable" expression of the wine's character through fruit, tannin, acidity, balance—terroir—is considered and discussed along with the wine's relation to the human element, as part of the full gustatory and, I would add, intellectual and emotional experience, of wine.

. . . .

BAINBRIDGE ISLAND VINEYARDS & WINERY
SS
989 N.E. Day Road · Bainbridge Island, WA 98110
(206) 842-9463 · www.bainbridgevineyards.com

For years, Gerard and Jo Ann Bentryn bucked the system, growing cool-climate grapes such as Müller-Thurgau, Siegerrebe, and Madeleine Angevine organically on rainy Bainbridge Island. The couple built a beautiful little vineyard and tasting room, and now, for health reasons, are passing the winery on to new owners (hopefully). But their dedication to sustainability and their awareness of the interconnectedness of food, wine, agriculture, wildlife, and the land will continue to influence those whom they came into contact with in the wine business. At the time of this writing, Bainbridge Island Vineyards & Winery's future is uncertain, but with any luck, the Bentryns' legacy will carry on in the form of new ownership as dedicated to sustainable winegrowing as they were.

BUTY WINERY
SS (Conner Lee Chardonnay)
35 E. Cessna Avenue · Walla Walla, WA 99362
(509) 527-0901 · www.butywinery.com

Buty Winery has long relied on sourcing great fruit from vineyards in the Walla Walla and Yakima Valleys. For owner Nina Buty Foster, finding the purest expression of each vineyard's fruit helped create "focused blends of Cabernet Sauvignon and Syrah." A new estate vineyard, called Rockgarden, is planted in the highest 5 percent elevation of "The Rocks," a cobblestone-covered area south of Walla Walla near Milton-Freewater, Oregon. An old apple orchard was prepared organically, and vines were planted densely in Syrah, Cabernet Sauvignon, Grenache, Mourvèdre, Marsanne, and Roussanne. This vineyard should be in production of certified-organic fruit, grown especially for Buty's signature Rediviva of the Stones red blend, in 2012. Buty has long sourced fruit from Washington's best wineries, some certified Salmon-Safe, LIVE, and working toward organic certification. Phinny Hill Vineyard, for example, is working toward organic certification, and Conner Lee Vineyard is certified Salmon-Safe.

CAYUSE VINEYARDS
17 E. Main Street · Walla Walla, WA 99362
(509) 526-0686 · www.cayusevineyards.com
Biodynamic practices

The first certified-biodynamic vineyards in the state are also producing some of the most sought-after wines. Christophe Baron's Cayuse Vineyards, first planted in Walla Walla in 1997, is pushing into new (and old) territory with its plantings. Baron had a life-changing experience when he first visited from France and saw the stony fields south of Walla Walla that would become his vineyards. He likened the fields of round stones left by the Missoula Floods to the great old vineyards full of *galets roulés*, or rolled, round cobbles, in the southern Rhône in France. Plowing and planting these unyielding fields, he came by his "Crazy Frenchman" moniker honestly, ignoring people's criticism that he'd "break his equipment and waste his money." Baron didn't care. He adopted some of the methods his winegrowing family in Champagne had used, including using draft horses to plow and planting vines extremely close together—in his latest plantings the vines bump right up against each other. In general, Baron goes far "beyond organic" in his respect for his land. "Mistreating the earth kills the terroir," he insists, "and you end up with soils that are sick or dead. [Soil] is a foundation you have to protect."

Wines to Try: Cayuse is well known for its Bionic Frog Syrah, a nod to Christophe Baron's Frenchness and his endless energy. This is always a bold wine, with complexity and layers of aromas and flavors of smoke, meat, black plum, cardamom, and licorice. Voluptuously graceful and full of fine tannins, his wines display the fresh acidity Washington is known for, with the purity of fruit reflecting the uniqueness of Cayuse's terroir.

CHATEAU STE. MICHELLE
LIVE · SS
14111 N.E. 145th Street · Woodinville, WA 98072
(425) 488-1133 · www.ste-michelle.com

Washington's largest winery owns about 3,500 vineyard acres across the state and contracts with many other growers as well, but only in the past few years has sustainability become a watchword. In 2009, two of Chateau Ste. Michelle's top vineyards, Cold Creek (about 700 acres), in the Columbia Valley AVA, and Canoe Ridge (about 550 acres), in the Horse Heaven Hills AVA, have gone through the process of becoming LIVE certified and Salmon-Safe. Chateau Ste. Michelle has been a leader in education and viticulture since the 1970s, and hopefully its interest in certifying vineyards and reducing energy and water consumption will continue and grow. These two vineyards have implemented a host of practices, including the planting of beneficial cover crops; controlled spraying of "soft" pesticides such as biodegradable oils, soaps, and plant extracts; using manure from local dairy operations, as well as pomace from winemaking in their compost; and installing drip irrigation systems. In the winery, fixtures, compressors, waste pond pumps, and refrigeration units have been replaced, cutting electrical usage in 2011 by 9.5 percent. In January 2010, it installed a new heat exchanger, which warms up the wine before bottling. And water is recycled, reducing consumption by almost 100 percent over that of the previous system. Chateau Ste. Michelle also recycled 128 tons of glass, metal, plastic, wood, paper, and cardboard in 2011, up from 102 tons in 2010.

CHINA BEND WINERY
CO

3751 Vineyard Way · Kettle Falls, WA 99141
(509) 732-6123 · www.chinabend.com

Winemaking is only part of what China Bend is up to. In addition to a certified-organic vineyard, proprietor Bart Alexander has gardens, a bed-and-breakfast, and a tasting room on the shore of Lake Roosevelt in northeastern Washington. China Bend's wines have no sulfites and are vegan, meaning they don't use eggs or isinglass for fining. While it's true that it has been making wine since the days when organic wine had a reputation for not tasting that great, some of its estate-grown wines suited to this cooler climate, such as Marechal Foch or the Alsatian red variety Léon Millot, are worth a second look. At China Bend, you can enjoy delicious food and wine in a beautiful setting, knowing that the food and the wines are fully organic. It also sells other foods, including organic jams, pickles, salsa, and coffee roasted at the winery.

CLAAR CELLARS
LIVE · SS
1001 Vintage Valley Parkway · Zillah, WA 98953
(509) 829-6810 · www.claarcellars.com

Claar Cellars had been selling grapes to wineries in Washington and other states for years, ever since Audrienne and Russell Claar planted their first grapes in 1980 on the family farm they'd owned since 1950, above steep cliffs on the Columbia River. Their daughter, Crista Claar Whitelatch, and her husband, Bob, were instrumental in starting to produce Claar Cellars' own wines in 1997. They make estate-grown Chardonnay, Sauvignon Blanc, Merlot, and Cabernet Sauvignon from grapes grown on their 120-acre White Bluffs Vineyard, which is LIVE and Salmon-Safe certified. In 2012 the winery facility also earned these two certifications.

DUNHAM CELLARS
LIVE (Double River) · SS (Double River and Frenchtown Vineyards)
150 E. Boeing Avenue · Walla Walla, WA 99362
(509) 529-4685 · www.dunhamcellars.com

Over the years, Dunham Cellars has gone from sourcing some of the best fruit in the state (which it still does) to growing its own. Vineyard manager Ken Hart is well known in Washington for his wisdom in these matters, planting Pepper Bridge Vineyard in 1991 and Seven Hills Vineyard in 1997. Now, for Dunham, he manages the Double River and Frenchtown Vineyards as well as the Lewis Estate Vineyard. His goal is to make "only a positive impact on the ecosystem," and he evaluates any inputs to make sure they will only affect the microbial balance in the soil in a positive way.

FIGGINS FAMILY WINE ESTATES / LEONETTI CELLAR
LIVE · SS
1859 Foothills Lane · Walla Walla, WA 99362
(509) 526-8040 · www.figginsfamily.com

"Tasting our wine is like looking into a mirror," says Leonetti and Figgins winemaker Chris Figgins. "The wine wasn't born on the crush pad; it originated months earlier when the season began, and, in fact, even years before that, when planting, trellising, spacing, and varietal decisions were made." His father, winemaker Gary Figgins, and his mother, Nancy, put Leonetti Winery on the map in 1977 as Walla Walla's first bonded winery, and they continue to make intense red wines that have achieved cult status. Enter the next generation: Chris grew up in the winery and notes the influence of Leonetti's very first wine, a 1978 White Riesling, on his wine education. Chris has taken Leonetti Cellar to the next level and has also started his own label, Figgins; both labels are now made from 100 percent estate-grown grapes, farmed according to sustainable Vinea practices. Chris has also taken the concept of terroir to the Figgins family ranch, the Lostine Cattle Company, whose herd of Highland cattle is completely pasture-raised without antibiotics or hormones. Sometimes they're even fed a treat of pomace from the famous wineries—now *that's* terroir.

Wines to Try: The heavenly Sangiovese, with its characteristically bright acidity, silky tannins, and long finish, shows how beautiful a Washington Sangiovese can be in the right vineyard, in the right hands. These wines are sold only through mailing (and waiting) lists, which you can join online.

GILBERT CELLARS
Not certified
5 N. Front Street · Yakima, WA 98901
(509) 249-9049 · www.gilbertcellars.com

For the Gilbert Family, sustainability is more than a recent development. This five-generation farming family has changed and grown over the past 100-plus years, since H. M. Gilbert moved his family from Illinois to start growing apples in Yakima's Ahtanum Valley. "We are able to make decisions for the long term, and all decisions are made with the idea that we're preserving the family heritage and property for future generations," says general manager Jessica Moskwa. "Intergenerational expertise informs our decisions in the vineyard, helping us balance tradition and innovation." The Gilberts acquired many orchards and vineyards, including the organic Doc Stewart Vineyard, planted in 1972. One of the largest organic fruit growers in the state, they use a "soft" spray program, spraying organic applications only when needed and following the LIVE protocol, although they are not certified. The Doc Stewart Vineyard, in the Wahluke Slope, is surrounded by an array of other fruit (apples, nectarines, and cherries), supporting biodiversity beneficial to insects and other fauna in the area.

HEDGES FAMILY ESTATE WINERY
DB (estate vineyard)
1859 Foothills Lane · Walla Walla, WA 99362
(509) 526-8040 · www.hedgesfamilyestate.com

One of the largest family-owned wineries in the state, Hedges is truly a family affair. Tom and Anne-Marie started their winery in 1987 and eventually built an estate winery on Red Mountain. They raised their children right: Son Christophe is a passionate rogue in marketing Hedges wines, refusing to enter into the ratings game and designing their gorgeous and amusing labels to suggest an ancient family legacy. They have a small estate winery that is farmed biodynamically and whose grapes are used in their wines, but they also acquire grapes from other vineyards. Daughter Sarah Hedges Goedhart is assistant winemaker to Tom's brother Pete Hedges. Sarah and her husband, Brent, have their own award-winning label, Goedhart Family Winery, and Pete and Sarah are also the winemakers for Obelisco Estate winery.

Wines to Try: With a focus on Red Mountain terroir, the Hedges Red Mountain Red Blend, with varying amounts of Cabernet Sauvignon and Merlot each year, is lush and ripe, with black fruits, coffee, and cocoa notes, and with the acidity and tannins necessary for long life.

HIGHTOWER CELLARS
LEED
19418 E. 583 PR N.E. · Benton City, WA 99320
(509) 588-2867 · www.hightowercellars.com

One way wineries are changing the way they do business is in the production facility itself. Tim and Kelly Hightower started their winery in 1997 in a nondescript warehouse space in Woodinville. Eventually they purchased a vineyard site on Red Mountain and built a winery in the available buildings. As the operation grew, they finally got to the point where they could renovate the winery and tasting room, and decided to do it according to LEED standards. So they hired Joe Chauncey, LEED architect at the Boxwood Design firm, who educated them about the issues surrounding sustainable wineries. "According to the US Green Building Council," says Chauncey, "building construction and demolition add 136 million tons of waste to US landfills each year. An old brick building on Main Street, an unused barn, and small, older warehouses have all been successfully transformed into working wineries through thoughtful adaptive reuse and are helping to reduce this number." He advised the Hightowers to, instead of building a new facility, renovate an old stable into a one-room facility with an outdoor patio where they can do everything from crush to bottling. He designed a *brise soleil*, or sunscreen, to shade the walls and lower cooling needs inside the winery. They also installed recycled barrel staves on the exterior—a beautiful addition to a winery that reflects the vision and quality of the excellent wines produced by this dynamic couple.

HOLLYWOOD HILL VINEYARDS
Not certified
14366 Woodinville-Redmond Road · Redmond, WA 98052
(425) 405-5799 · www.hollywoodhillvineyards.com

In a bold move, winegrower Steve Snyder of Hollywood Hill Vineyards started a vineyard of Pinot Noir and Chardonnay in Woodinville, on the west side (or·"wet side") of the Cascade Range. He says, "Eastern Washington is unique in that it's so dry; many vineyards hardly have to be sprayed. But here on the west side we battle rots and fungus. We're working with many new hybridized grapes that hardly have to be sprayed with any chemicals." He also grows other cool-climate grapes and sells cuttings of Zweigelt, St. Laurent, Garanoir, Dornfelder, Regent, Auxerrois, Sauvignon Blanc, Pinot Gris, Pinot Blanc, and Pinot Meunier. He sources most of his grapes from some of the dry side's best vineyards, two of which are grown organically: Portteus (certified organic and Salmon-Safe) and Gilbert (not certifed).

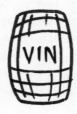

- -

JOY ANDERSON: WINERYWISE WINEMAKER

When Joy Anderson started making wine in 1981, after earning a chemistry degree and then doing fruit research for the USDA, she was working at Chateau Ste. Michelle at a time when there were only 24 winemakers in Washington State. Furthermore, she was one of just a few women in the field. The state's industry has now grown to 750 wineries, and many women thrive in it. Anderson is humble about her accomplishments, but she has quietly been making changes that have redirected the entire industry toward sustainable winegrowing and winemaking practices.

This is impressive in itself. But for many years she also happened to be one of the few winemakers creating really tasty organic wines in Washington. Now, at Snoqualmie Winery, Anderson is developing a program for the Washington Association of Wine Grape Growers called Winerywise, a program of self-evaluations, checklists, and action plans for wineries wanting to become more sustainable. Her vital work in the area of sustainability is now being recognized, as consumers grow more interested in where their wine comes from and how it is produced. Joy Anderson is the go-to expert, and her work is finally paying off in a market that wants purer wine with a conscience.

- -

L'ECOLE No. 41
SS · VINEA
41 Lowden School Road · Lowden, WA 99362
(509) 525-0940 · www.lecole.com

Winemaker Marty Clubb has seen the Walla Walla Valley wine industry grow from a few vineyards among wheat fields and orchards to 160-plus wineries throughout this beautiful valley's golden rolling hills. Clubb's complex, elegant reds and refreshing Old World–style whites are sourced from Pepper Bridge Vineyard, L'Ecole's estate vineyards (Seven Hills and Ferguson Ridge), and other vineyards in Walla Walla, as well as vineyards throughout the Columbia Valley. "All our Walla Walla Valley wines come from Vinea Certified Sustainable vineyards, a program that was influenced by Oregon's LIVE certification program," Clubb says. "We want to show the specific attributes of the vineyards, and it is easier to produce sustainable wines in the Walla Walla Valley than the rest of the Columbia Valley, because vineyards in this area were early adopters of sustainable certification." But Clubb suggests that many Washington growers are lucky in that the pressures from mildew, fungus, and pests is lower than for their neighbors to the wetter, cooler south in Oregon. In general, Washington vineyards don't have to use as much, or as many, chemicals. But there are other issues in Washington's dry climate, such as water usage, since, without irrigation, 99 percent of the vineyards in the state couldn't exist. Sourcing from many vineyards across a broad agricultural area brings up a complex set of decisions when it comes to sustainable farming. L'Ecole No. 41 has been navigating this territory and making great choices for 20-plus years and two generations and is looking ahead to a long, sustainable future.

Wines to Try: It is not often you come across a great white Bordeaux-style blend in the United States, but there are a few gems, and L'Ecole No. 41's Estate Luminesce is one of them. Sémillon-heavy, showing the stone fruit lushness balanced with the bright lime zest of Sauvignon Blanc. From year to year, one of my favorites. The Apogee Red Blend is also consistently excellent, and with fruit from Pepper Bridge Vineyard, you can't go wrong. The latest is a layered blend of Cabernet Sauvignon, Merlot, Malbec, and Cabernet Franc, with black plums, spice and leather, cocoa, good tannin structure, and bright acidity.

LEONETTI CELLAR (see Figgins Family Wine Estates)

LOPEZ ISLAND VINEYARDS AND WINERY
CO · SS
724 Fisherman Bay Road · Lopez Island, WA 98261
(360) 468-3644 · www.lopezislandvineyards.com

Brent Charnley is truly a pioneer in Washington wine, building the only winery on Lopez Island, one of two estate wineries in the San Juan Islands. But more than that, Charnley's deep commitment to "local, sustainable, low environmental impact, and human health values" is a model for others. And Charnley has created a vineyard that works within the particular ecosystem of Lopez Island (the driest of the San Juans), growing certified-organic and Salmon-Safe grapes that thrive in this cool maritime climate. His unusual varieties, Madeline Angevine, from the Loire Valley in France, and the German Siegerrebe, a cross between Madeleine Angevine and Gewürztraminer, are two aromatic white grapes that make lovely, floral wines full of stone fruit aromas and flavors. Charnley also makes excellent red wines, some from organically grown grapes from the Yakima Valley, as well as fruit wines from island orchards.

Wines to Try: Brent Charnley's wines go exceptionally well with food. The Siegerrebe is made in an off-dry style, which is a perfect match for the fresh spice of Thai or Vietnamese food. The Madeleine is in a dry style, perfect with Lopez Island clams or oysters.

MEMALOOSE
Not certified
34 State Street · Lyle, WA 98635
(360) 635-2887 · www.winesofthegorge.com

Brian McCormick and his father, Rob, tend vineyards on each side of the Columbia River, overlooking the steep cliffs and mountains of the Columbia Gorge AVA. Brian makes "wines for food," which are crafted in a more Old World style, with lower alcohol and higher acidity than many big, fruity, high-alcohol wines of the New World. Of his five vineyards, Hannah's Bench and Hamm's Vineyard are farmed sustainably, and Parker's Vineyard, the Annex, and Idiot's Grace Vineyard are farmed organically. They produce a beautiful Cabernet Franc and an off-dry Riesling that indeed are excellent food wines. McCormick sees the Gorge AVA as "America's most unique winegrowing region," for its steep cliffs, hot days and cool nights, and amazing views. Its amazing array of microclimates, with elevations from 50 to 2,000 feet, its cloud cover, rain, and soils (from volcanic to loess), means that almost any grape variety can grow there, and McCormick has planted more than a dozen varieties, from Grenache to Primitivo and Sangiovese.

Wines to Try: A beautifully aromatic wine, Trevitt's White is a blend of Viognier, Roussanne, Marsanne, and Muscat. Evoking white flowers and white peach, with zesty citrus, this wine always has superb acidity and accompanies pork and poultry beautifully.

NACHES HEIGHTS VINEYARD·
SS
2410 Naches Heights Road · Yakima, WA 98908
(855) 648-9463 · www.nhvines.com

Phil Cline is building a bit of a dynasty on the Naches Heights plateau. It's an area few have heard of, but it was recently named Washington's 12th American Viticultural Area. Cline grew up on his parents' orchard in Naches Heights, a farming community above the town of Yakima, in an area that ranges in elevation from 1,200 to 2,100 feet and has soils from pre–Missoula Floods volcanic activity called the Goat Rocks lava flow. Naches Heights Vineyard sits at 1,680 feet, making this one of the highest-elevation vineyard sites in Washington, and it is farmed organically and biodynamically, although only certified LIVE and Salmon-Safe at present. Cline also manages the Wilridge Vineyard for Paul Beveridge of Wilridge Winery and Aecetia Vineyards, owned by his neighbor David McKinnon, both of which are Demeter Certified Biodynamic. Aecetia fruit will soon be used in Naches Heights wines. Cool-climate grapes such as Pinot Gris, Riesling, and Gewürztraminer grow here. Syrah, Tempranillo, and Albariño are planted, making for some very interesting wines. The Aecetia Vineyard property boasts a beautiful new tasting room and gardens.

NOVELTY HILL/JANUIK WINERY
SS (Stillwater Creek Estate Wines, Seven Hills Cabernet Sauvignon)
14710 Woodinville-Redmond Road N.E. · Woodinville, WA 98072
(425) 481-5502 · www.noveltyhilljanuik.com

Novelty Hill and Januik Wineries are part of a partnership between former Chateau Ste. Michelle winemaker Mike Januik and partners Tom Alberg and Judi Beck. The wines are made from grapes grown in Stillwater Creek Vineyard, one of the steepest sites in Washington, a south-facing, 245-acre vineyard on the Royal Slope of the Frenchman Hills, with a 22 percent grade in places. While that means the drainage is great, if pesticides and herbicides were applied, they too would easily drain off this large vineyard and into surface water that eventually ends up in the Columbia River a few miles away. In 2007, Stillwater Creek Vineyard became the first Columbia Valley vineyard to be certified Salmon-Safe; Januik also sources from some of the best vineyards across the state, including another Salmon-Safe vineyard, Seven Hills Vineyard. Stillwater Creek wines have great natural acidity, due to the climate in this special vineyard: It is sunny 300 days a year, but temperatures, usually in the 80s in the summer, can drop by 30–40 degrees at night.

PACIFIC RIM
DB
West Richland, WA
(800) 818-7979 · www.rieslingrules.com
No tasting room

The first certified-biodynamic vineyard in Washington was the Wallula Vineyard, high on the cliffs above the Columbia River at Wallula Gap, where the famous series of Missoula Floods were blocked from flowing any farther about 12,000 to 18,000 years ago, before spilling into the Columbia River. The fruit from this vineyard goes into Pacific Rim's 10 or so delicious Riesling wines, from bone dry to dessert sweet. The only certified-organic and -biodynamic vineyard in the state, Wallula is a model for other vineyards that are moving in this direction, with prominent educational information in all its marketing pieces, in which it emphasizes the need to "walk the walk" and not take part in corporate greenwashing. The whole-farm idea is in full force at the 160-acre Wallula Vineyard, with sustainable practices as part of the winery's mission to make "pure" wine. No chemical fertilizers, pesticides, or herbicides are used, nor commercial yeasts in the winery. Sheep, nature's most diligent weed killer, wander the rows, keeping grass and weeds down. Pacific Rim is also committed to saving water and energy and uses low-weight, 50 percent recycled bottles that lower CO_2 emissions by 33 percent and allow for 25 percent more bottles per truck. It has partnered with the Wild Salmon Center (www.wildsalmoncenter.org) in a promotion called Save Water, Drink Riesling, to bring more donations to the center. With the intense commitment to biodynamics and humor, it's no surprise that this winery was first a project of Bonny Doon Vineyards' Randall Grahm. He sold the winery in 2011 to Banfi Vintners, which is owned by the Mariani family in New York, and they vow to keep it a Riesling-focused winery with a commitment to sustainability.

Wines to Try: Start with the Demeter Certified Biodynamic Rieslings from Wallula Vineyard. These wines are just pretty, with heady aromatics of jasmine and grapefruit, tropical fruit, and lime. A bright minerality and acidity even in the riper years give these wines a clean flavor that reflects the care taken in the winery and vineyards. The website lists the ingredients in these wines: biodynamic grapes, sulfites below 100 ppm, yeast hulls, and bentonite (used for protein stability), showing a dedication to the "truest form of Riesling."

PEPPER BRIDGE
LIVE · SS · VINEA
14810 N.E. 145th Street · Woodinville, WA 98072
(425) 483-7026 · www.pepperbridge.com

Norm McKibben planted his first vineyard south of Walla Walla and started Pepper Bridge Winery with partner Ray Goff in 1998. He has been at the vortex of the exponential growth in Washington wine ever since. An innovator dedicated to making winegrowing more environmentally friendly and his business more efficient and sustainable, McKibben introduced several new technologies to grape growing, including state-of-the-art irrigation systems that deliver not only water but compost teas to just the right spots at just the right amounts in the vineyard. His soil moisture and temperature monitoring equipment notifies the crew via their smartphones when moisture is detected below the roots or in other areas of the vineyard, helping Pepper Bridge to conserve water and not overwater their vines. Two estate vineyards are LIVE and Salmon-Safe certified: Pepper Bridge, which has grown from 10 to 200 acres of Cabernet Franc, Cabernet Sauvignon, Malbec, Merlot, Petit Verdot, Sangiovese, and Syrah; and Seven Hills, managed by Chris Banek, which supplies some of Washington's best wineries with Cabernet Franc, Cabernet Sauvignon, Carménère,

Grenache, Malbec, Merlot, Petit Verdot, Sangiovese, Sauvignon Blanc, Sémillon, and Syrah. Seven Hills was recognized by *Wine&Spirits* magazine in 2004 as one of the 10 great vineyards of the world. Pepper Bridge's winery makes very few wines: a Merlot, a Cabernet Sauvignon, the Trine red blend, and a Reserve red blend, all from the estate vineyards south of the town of Walla Walla and just north of the Oregon border. Winemaker Jean-François Pellet's attention to detail is evident in the vineyard, for instance, encouraging wild roses and blackberries as habitat for a parasitic wasp that controls leafhoppers. The winery has also switched to softer organic products over harsh chemicals to control powdery mildew.

SNOQUALMIE VINEYARDS
CO
60 Frontier Road · Prosser, WA 99350
(509) 786-5558 · www.snoqualmie.com

Winemaker Joy Anderson says that in winemaking, it's best to leave Mother Nature alone, and she has been doing that since 1991 in one of the state's few certified-organic wineries. Snoqualmie has the largest number of certified-organic vineyards—378 acres—in the state, with another 149 acres in the process of certification. Its 2010 "Sustainability and Organics Report" (it publishes them online every year since 2007, something that should be part of every winery's sustainable approach) states that the winery lowered both its electricity and water usage by about 30 percent, mostly through employee education and awareness training and fixing air leaks in compressors. The industry standard is 2.9 gallons of water used for each gallon of wine produced; Snoqualmie used 2.834 gallons, down from 4.263 gallons, with a goal of 2.3 gallons. It will be reusing gray water and using closed system jackets to heat and cool the wine without using water. Snoqualmie is definitely a leader in becoming more sustainable, not only in its methods but in its educational events, including the "Greener Living and Harvest Celebration," which brings together organic vendors, organic food, and wine pairings; it drew 300 people in 2008.

Wines to Try: Known for Riesling, Snoqualmie also was one of the first wineries to make "naked" Chardonnay, keeping it in stainless steel tanks rather than oak barrels, to show off the true fruit character of the grape. This dry, apple-and-pear (and mineral) wine is super-versatile, pairing with poultry and salads, cheeses and charcuterie.

SPOILED DOG WINERY
Not certified
5881 Maxwelton Road · Langley, WA 98260
(360) 661-6226 · www.spoileddogwinery.com

You have to hand it to the courageous people who try to grow wine grapes in the islands of Puget Sound. Jack and Karen Krug run one of the few wineries making estate-grown Pinot Noir in Washington. What's more, their wine has been gaining acclaim: Their 2009 Pinot won a double gold at the Seattle Wine Awards. The Whidbey Island maritime climate suits these cool-weather grapes, and the Krugs' attitude toward farming shows a solid commitment to sustainability. Not just a vineyard, but a working farm producing apples, pears, and grass-fed Black Angus cattle, Spoiled Dog uses "best practices" organic and biodynamic methods but is not certified. The Krugs use llama and cow manure in compost, manage weeds mechanically rather than with herbicides, and credit their dogs with keeping pests and grape-eating birds out of the vineyard. Rain barrels collect some of that northwest sunshine to use for keeping the cows hydrated. An apple-pear wine called Pomo di Moro is made with fruit from the farm, and the Krugs also make a rosé blend of Pinot Noir and Pinot Gris. A sense of fun is another important part of this farm, with a "Spoiled Dog Contest" each year. This year's winner was a whole crop of dachshunds; maybe their prize could be a week on the farm visiting with the two resident spoiled dogs, Blue and Sami, and chasing off gophers.

TERRA BLANCA WINERY & ESTATE VINEYARD
SS
34715 N. Demoss Road · Benton City, WA 99320
(509) 588-6082 · www.terrablanca.com

Terra Blanca's 91-acre vineyard is situated on a 300-acre parcel near the Yakima River on an old riverbed composed of fine, sandy silt loams with interbeds of carbonate-coated gravels, cobbles, and boulders. The vineyard soil holds very little water, so drip irrigation is tightly controlled. Winemaker Keith Pilgrim feels that this dry, well-drained site "develops better intrinsic strength for fighting harmful bacteria, illnesses, and fungi." Basically carved out of a steep hillside covered with native sagebrush and balsamroot flowers, the area wouldn't sustain much else without irrigation. Many winegrowers love this area because of that; the judicious use of water helps to control fungus, vigorous leaf growth, and weeds.

TWO MOUNTAIN WINERY
Not certified
2151 Cheyne Road · Zillah, WA 98953
(509) 829-3900 · www.twomountainwinery.com

Matt and Patrick Rawn are part of a farming family that has been growing peaches, apricots, prunes, and apples in the Yakima Valley for 50 years. They have seen the industry transition from conventional farming to commercial certified-organic tree fruit practices, and they've witnessed the dramatic transition from fruit to vineyards in the state.

Their grandfather, Phil Schmidt, planted orchards in 1951, and uncle Ron Schmidt planted their estate Copeland Vineyard in 2000. "Pat and I noticed that there were high and low points to both disciplines [conventional and organic]," says winemaker Matt Rawn. Now they are combining what they've observed to create what they call low-impact farming, which they feel is more comprehensive and sustainable for the crop, the environment, and the workforce. As an example, the Rawns spray organically approved, inexpensive sulfur for powdery mildew (which is a big concern for wine grapes), until it becomes too hot and will hurt the crop. "We then use a systemic fungicide to control the mildew once we are in the heat of the summer until the grapes turn color. We use only two applications on the crop, limiting the amount of exposure to the applicator and surrounding environment, amount of fuel used, the amount of dust raised, expense, and the amount of soil compacted," Matt says. If they used the conventional method, they would apply fungicide much earlier and throughout the season; if they used only the organic method of spraying sulfur all season, they feel they would "run the risk of burning the leaves and berries and therefore hurt the quality of the end product." The Rawns feel this low-impact method is cheaper and safer than the way things were done when their grandfather planted his vineyard.

UPCHURCH VINEYARD
LIVE · SS
Kirkland, WA
www.upchurchvineyard.com
No tasting room

Chris Upchurch, longtime award-winning winemaker for DeLille Cellars, and his wife and partner, Theodora, recently planted a vineyard on Red Mountain. They consulted with one of the best, Dick Boushey, who has managed some of the state's best vineyards for decades. Upchurch was focused from the beginning on sustainability, receiving LIVE and Salmon-Safe certification early in the vineyard's life, working with a hot, dry, windy ecosystem that makes it easier to avoid herbicides, fungicides, and pesticides in the vineyard. At the time of this writing, the first wine from Upchurch Vineyard was settled in the cellar, waiting for the right time to be released.

WATERS
SS (Loess Syrah, Pepper Bridge Syrah) · VINEA
1825 J. B. George Road · Walla Walla, WA 99362
(509) 525-1514 · www.waterswinery.com

Waters Winery winemaker Jamie Brown is becoming known for creating wines that reflect the intriguing terroir of the Walla Walla Valley, especially from the estate's Forgotten Hills Vineyard, which Brown calls "a very, very challenging vineyard." At 950 feet in elevation, this cooler site ripens later than most of the area's vineyards, and "the whims of Mother Nature more often than not leave us with little of its truly spectacular fruit," he says. "In 2010, we did indeed get fruit, but it didn't offer the same characteristics that our 'FH devotees' look for every year. At the same time, our Old Stones vineyard produced some inspiring Grenache; however, not quite enough to be used solo. Thus, Waters has produced its first ever Syrah blend: 92 percent Syrah and 8 percent Grenache, all aged in neutral oak." This manner of pulling flavors from what the vineyard provides results in some incredibly interesting wines. They may never be as popular as the riper, fuller-bodied Syrah and Cabernet Sauvignon Waters is known for, but the dried herb and floral, smoke and slatey notes make wines like this worth trying, if only to savor while contemplating the elusive concept of terroir. On the winery side, Waters has received attention for its energy-efficient and progressive design. The designer, LEED architect Joe

Chauncey of Boxwood Design, also designed other wine-related projects, including Col Solare on Red Mountain, Hightower Winery, the Northwest Wine Academy in Seattle, and the Carlton Winemakers Studio in Oregon. At Waters, materials used include reclaimed corrugated metal and wood, which fit into the agricultural landscape with a contemporary flair. A skylight in the barrel room reduces the need for electric light, and the rooms are arranged to protect the barrel room from the intense afternoon heat.

Wines to Try: The Waters' Loess Vineyard Syrah is from Leonetti's Estate Vineyard and shows an amazing range of aromatics. It is co-fermented with a small amount of Viognier as done in the northern Rhône to brighten the deep, dark red with intriguing aromas of violets, rose, and truffle, fine tannins and soft acidity, black fruits and dark chocolate flavors. This is a special wine to enjoy with herb-grilled meats.

WILRIDGE WINERY
DB
1416 34th Avenue · Seattle, WA 98122
(206) 325-3051 · www.wilridgewinery.com

The fullest expression of biodynamic viniculture in Washington State, the 85 acres of Wilridge Vineyard are farmed biodynamically by owner Paul Beveridge and vineyard manager Phil Cline (see sidebar, "Paul Beveridge and Phil Cline: A Biodynamic Partnership"), who is also the owner and winemaker for Naches Heights Vineyard. Wilridge Vineyard started as an experiment by Beveridge, who felt that some of the best wines in the world are farmed biodynamically and wanted to see how it worked with this new site, planted in 2007. For 20 years before planting the vineyard, Beveridge purchased grapes from vineyards all over the state. He still uses grapes from certain sites to fill in areas of winemaking that he can't produce from his vineyard—for instance, the deep, rich, bold reds from Klipsun Vineyard on Red Mountain.

Wines to Try: The Wilridge Nebbiolo is a beautiful example of biodynamics at work. Delicately aromatic but boldly flavored, this wine shows a purity of fruit with its bright cherry and roses, with bright acidity and intense but still silky tannins that will help this wine age well.

WOODWARD CANYON
LIVE · SS · VINEA
1920 W. Highway 12 · Lowden, WA 99360
(509) 525-4129 · www.woodwardcanyon.com

Rick Small and Darcey Fugman-Small are pretty busy people and very involved in transforming the wine industry into a more sustainable business. They are founding members of Vinea, and Woodward Canyon is also LIVE and Salmon-Safe certified in its estate vineyard. "We prefer to focus on sustainability," says Rick, "even though we may pursue organic farming and green practices, because sustainability looks at the overall operation, the environmental, social, and economic systems. In sustainable terms, this means we are dealing with a triple bottom line: economic (making a profit), environmental (minimal and safe chemical use), and social (being a good neighbor and employer)." The couple is involved with ReCORK, a cork recycling program (see sidebar, "Put a Cork in It," in the Sustainability in the Winery chapter) that gathers corks at drop-off sites across the United States then grinds and reuses the cork material for footwear and packaging. Woodward Canyon's tasting room garden was planted on an area that had been used for livestock around an old farmhouse, and there were "no worms in the soil, no songbirds or wildlife." After a few years of building the soil, planting plants that attract beneficial insects, things have changed: Now quail, hawks, killdeer, rabbits, and butterflies enjoy the garden. Rick Small suggests that if a winery claims to be "green" or "sustainable," you should try to find out more. "Ask if they are members of an organic or sustainable certifying organization," he suggests. "Ask what, specifically, they are doing in the winery and/or vineyard and how long they have been doing it." Rick and Darcey and their crew add new elements to their sustainability picture every year, including energy saving in the winery and lighter bottles for their excellent wines.

PAUL BEVERIDGE AND PHIL CLINE: A BIODYNAMIC PARTNERSHIP

An attorney by trade and *garagiste* winemaker of Wilridge Winery by avocation, Paul Beveridge turned his focus toward farming his own wine grapes in 2007. He hired vineyard manager Phil Cline to plant his vineyards in an unexplored region of the Yakima Valley near Cline's vineyard and family orchards, from which he had been buying fruit for years. Naches Heights is a 1,800-foot-elevation plateau in the foothills of the Cascade Range, above the areas affected by the Missoula Floods, with topsoils of 100 percent windblown loess—the finest topsoil in the world, according to Beveridge. The vineyard is situated west of Yakima, among 100-year-old orchards. Cline and Beveridge decided to experiment on the 85-acre site and planted 22 varieties of grapes, from Pinot Gris to Nebbiolo, Sangiovese to Syrah, Cabernet Sauvignon, Souzão, Tinta Cão, Touriga Nacional, and Tempranillo.

They also decided to farm biodynamically. Phil was always a country boy, albeit an eccentric one, with his "rosé"-colored glasses and shock of wild red hair. Paul transitioned from city mouse to country mouse; more suntan, less stress.

For Beveridge, there was "never a question about farming organically," because he planned to spend a lot of time in the vineyard with his wife and young sons. Beveridge and Cline studied Rudolph Steiner's writings, which led to Goethe's writings on form and color, and to Nicolas Joly, the eccentric French evangelist of biodynamic farming. As the vineyard developed, and he began to make unmanipulated wines from grapes that had never seen chemicals, had been planted and harvested by seasonal cycles, and had been composted and sprayed with a wave of natural preparations, including homeopathically dosed teas of dandelion, stinging nettle, valerian, horsetail, silica, manure compost, and more, Beveridge began to see a change in the wines. "I am by nature a rational person and somewhat skeptical of the spiritual claims that underlie biodynamics," he says. "However, one cannot argue with the results—some of the best wines in the world come from biodynamic vineyards." And he is fully behind the idea of seeing the farm as a complete, self-sufficient unit.

On the cliffs above the historic Cowiche (*cow-witch-ee*) Canyon nature preserve, visitors can hike and ride bikes down from the vineyard and bask in the rugged beauty of these cliffs. Thanks to the perseverence (and paperwork) of Beveridge and Cline, Naches Heights was designated Washington's 12th American Viticultural Area. With their tasting room created from an old farmhouse, and absolutely beautiful, aromatic, and complex wines coming from Wilridge Vineyard, Beveridge and Cline's biodynamic experiment is in full bloom.

• •

OTHER WASHINGTON WINERIES WITH GREEN CONSIDERATIONS

ARBOR CREST WINE CELLARS
4705 N. Fruit Hill Road
Spokane, WA 99217
(509) 927-9463
Tasting room:
808 W. Main Avenue
Spokane, WA 99201
(509) 747-3903
SS (Conner Lee Chardonnay,
Cabernet Franc)

BAER WINERY
9501 144th Avenue
N.E. Woodinville, WA 98072
(425) 483-7060
www.baerwinery.com
SS

BERESAN WINERY
169 Peppers Bridge Road
Walla Walla, WA 99362
(509) 522-2395
www.beresanwines.com
SS.(Cabernet Franc, Cabernet
Sauvignon, Syrah)

BOOKWALTER
894 Tulip Lane
Richland, WA 99352
(509) 627-5000
www.bookwalterwines.com
SS (Conner Lee Couplet)

CHELAN ESTATE WINERY
755 S. Lakeshore Road
Chelan, WA 98816
(509) 682-5454
www.chelanestatewinery.com
SS (Stillwater Creek Vineyard:
Cabernet Sauvignon, Red Wine,
Merlot)

CHINOOK WINERY
220 W. Wittkopf Loop
Prosser, WA 99350
(509) 786-2725
www.chinookwines.com
Eco-Glass

CÔTE BONNEVILLE
2641 Fordyce Road
Sunnyside, WA 98944
(509) 840-4596
www.cotebonneville.com
By appointment only
SS

COVINGTON CELLARS
18580 142nd Avenue N.E.
Woodinville, WA 98072
(425) 806-8636
www.covingtoncellars.com
SS (Seven Hills Syrah)

FIVE STAR CELLARS
840 N.E. C Street
Walla Walla, WA 99324
(509) 527-8400
www.fivestarcellars.com
SS (Cabernet, Malbec, and reserve
wines)

**GARRISON CREEK CELLARS
ESTATE VINEYARD AND
WINERY**
4153 Hood Road
Walla Walla, WA 99362
(509) 527-7377
www.garrisoncreekcellars.com

GORMAN WINERY
19501 144th Avenue N.E., #C500
Woodinville, WA 98072
(206) 351-0719
www.gormanwinery.com
SS (Conner Lee Big Sissy
Chardonnay)

GUARDIAN CELLARS
19501 144th Avenue N.E., #E600
Woodinville, WA 98072
www.guardiancellars.com
SS (Conner Lee Gunmetal,
Stillwater Creek Angel)

JM CELLARS
4404 137th Place N.E.
Woodinville, WA 98072
(425) 485-6508
www.jmcellars.com
SS

LATAH CREEK
3030 E. Indiana Avenue
Spokane Valley, WA 99216
(509) 926-0164
www.latahcreek.com
SS (Chardonnay)

LULLABY WINERY
Walla Walla, WA
(509) 386-1342
No tasting room

MARK RYAN WINERY
Woodinville tasting room:
14810 N.E. 145th Street,
Building A-1
Woodinville, WA 98072
(425) 398-5433
Walla Walla tasting room:
26 E. Main Street, Suite 1
Walla Walla, WA 99362

(509) 876-4577
www.markryanwinery.com
SS (Chardonnay, Pinot Noir)

MASQUERADE CELLARS
2001 Iowa Street
Bellingham, WA 98229
(360) 220-7072
www.masqueradewines.com
ReCORK dropoff

MATTHEWS CELLARS
16116 140th Place N.E.
Woodinville, WA 98072
(425) 487-9810
www.matthewscellars.com
SS (Stillwater Creek Sauvignon
Blanc, Columbia Valley Red Wine)

MERRY CELLARS
1300 N.E. Henley Court
Pullman, WA 99163
(509) 338-4699
www.merrycellars.com
SS (Stillwater Creek Merlot and
Syrah, Walla Walla Valley wines)

NORTHSTAR WINERY
736 J. B. George Road
Walla Walla, WA 99362
(509) 525-6100
www.northstarwinery.com
SS (estate vineyard)

NOTA BENE CELLARS
9320 15th Avenue S., Unit CC
Seattle, WA 98108
(206) 459-3185
www.notabenecellars.com
SS (Conner Lee Red Wine)

PORTTEUS
5201 Highland Drive
Zillah, WA 98953
(509) 829-6970
www.portteus.com
CO

REININGER WINERY
5858 Old Highway 12
Walla Walla, WA 99362
(509) 522-1994
SS (Walla Walla Valley wines,
Helix Stillwater Creek)

SAVIAH CELLARS
1979 J. B. George Road
Walla Walla, WA 99362
(509) 520-5166
www.saviahcellars.com
SS (Stillwater Creek Vineyard and
Walla Walla Valley wines)

SEVEN HILLS WINERY
212 N. 3rd Avenue
Walla Walla, WA 99362
(877) 777-7870
www.sevenhillswinery.com
SS (Seven Hills and McClellan
estate vineyards)

SYNCLINE
111 Balch Road
Lyle, WA 98635
(509) 365-4361
www.synclinewine.com
Biodynamic practices

TAGARIS WINERY
44 Tulip Lane
Richland, WA 99352
(509) 628-1619
www.tagariswines.com
CO (Michael Vineyards)

TAMARACK CELLARS
700 C Street
Walla Walla, WA 99362
(509) 526-3533
www.tamarackcellars.com
SS (DeBrul Vineyard Reserve)

TEMPUS CELLARS
1110 C Street
Walla Walla, WA 99362
(509) 270-0298
www.tempuscellars.com
SS (Seven Hills Merlot, Walla
Walla Valley Syrah)

TERTULIA CELLARS
1564 Whiteley Road
Walla Walla, WA 99362
(509) 525-5700
www.tertuliacellars.com
SS (Les Collines Walla Walla
Valley Syrah, Tempranillo)

TRILLIUM CREEK WINERY
17812 G Street
Home, WA 98349
(253) 884-5746
www.trilliumcreekwinery.com
Low-sulfite wines

VA PIANO VINEYARDS
1793 J. B. George Road
Walla Walla, WA 99362
(509) 529-0900
www.vapianovineyards.com

WESTPORT WINERY
1 S. Arbor Road
Aberdeen, WA 98520
www.westportwinery.org
SS (estate wines)

WOODINVILLE WINE CELLARS
17721 132nd Avenue N.E.
Woodinville, WA 98072
(425) 481-8860
www.woodinvillewine.com
SS (Indomitable)
Eco-Glass

IDAHO WINERIES

Wine grapes have been grown in Idaho since 1864, but the modern wine business is still in its infancy there. In 2002 there were just 11 wineries in the state; now there are 48, with 1,600 acres of grapes planted, producing some excellent wines, from refreshing, dry Rieslings to lush Chardonnays to rich Cabernet Sauvignons and Syrahs. The Snake River Valley, situated on the 43rd parallel, is Idaho's sole AVA, with elevations from 1,500 to 3,000 feet, similar to those in the high-mountain desert Rioja region of Spain. But grapes are also grown in the southwestern and northern regions of the state.

There are two certified-organic wineries in Idaho, and the owners of Bitner Winery hope it soon will become the state's first LIVE-certified winery. Idaho Wine Commission director Moya Shatz Dolsby sees a bright future for Idaho wine. "I am hoping Bitner Vineyards will pave the way for others to follow in LIVE certification," she says. It will be interesting to see the industry grow, especially since some of these early wineries are focusing on sustainable practices and will no doubt be models for vineyards and wineries to come.

3 HORSE RANCH VINEYARDS
CO
5900 Pearl Road · Eagle, ID 83616
(208) 863-6561 · www.3horseranchvineyards.com

For owners Gary and Martha Cunningham, organic farming was a no-brainer. Their home was just above the vineyards, and they didn't want to breathe in any of the chemicals that are used in conventional viniculture. They committed to coming up with other ways to deal with pests and weeds and found organics to be "the right way for us to grow our grapes and tend our vineyards." Cover crops are planted to encourage beneficial insects and push out weeds, and compost and mulching build soil health. In the winery, the Cunninghams take a hands-off approach, adding the bare minimum of sulfites, in order to "ensure stable and delicious wine."

Wines to Try: The Estate Pinot Gris, with its intense aromas of orange and tropical fruit, apple-like acidity, and softness on the finish, is a refreshing and flavorful organic wine, with minimal sulfites added.

BITNER VINEYARDS
LIVE
16645 Plum Road · Caldwell, ID 83607
(208) 899-7648 · www.bitnervineyards.com · www.pollination.com

Bitner Vineyards is slated to become the first LIVE-certified vineyard in Idaho, but then, owners Ron and Mary Bitner have always been pioneers in the Snake River Valley. An entomologist by profession, Ron had the chance to travel the world consulting on bees and fell in love with Australian wine. He came back to Idaho to plant his first Riesling and Chardonnay vines in 1981. The Bitners sold grapes to Koenig Distillery and Winery for years, before starting to make their own wines in 1997. Currently the Intermountain Representative to the Wine America Board and president of the Wine Grape Growers of

America, Ron makes wines that capture the essence of the Snake River Valley terroir, which features high volcanic ash and old lake bottom sediment soils, in a dry, high-mountain desert climate. The property also includes a lovely bed-and-breakfast, a handy home base in the vineyards for winery tours.

CINDER
Not certified
107 E. 44th Street · Garden City, ID 83704
(208) 433-9813 · www.cinderwines.com

Winemaker Melanie Krause and her husband, Joe Schnerr, moved to Idaho with some plans. Melanie had been a winemaker at Chateau Ste. Michelle, learning the ropes, and she spent a summer visiting vineyards in the Snake River Valley AVA in Idaho in order to confirm her suspicion that this high-desert mountainous region was producing some world-class grapes. She found a fascinating terroir of volcanic soil, basalt, and cinders left from upwellings of magma through rifts that surround the valley and from the formation and receding of Ancient Lake Idaho, which at one point had reached a depth of 3,400 feet. When the lake receded, its bed was full of basalt and cinders that had erupted beneath the waters—hence the winery's name. Cinder sources from a range of vineyards in the area, including Williamson, Rocky Fence, Symms, Arena Valley, Skyline, and Sawtooth. Although there are few certified-organic or LIVE vineyards and wineries in Idaho, the hot, dry climate makes it easier to grow sustainably, and the influx of enthusiastic young people like Krause and Schnerr, who are dedicated to making wines that reflect the land and creating relationships with their local growers, will no doubt help transform Idaho's wine industry in coming decades.

HOLESINSKY CERTIFIED ORGANIC VINEYARD AND WINERY CO

4477 Valley Steppe Drive · Buhl, ID 83316
(208) 543-6940 · www.holesinsky.com

James Holesinsky's mission to create "world-class wine with no shortcuts, impurities, overprocessing, filtering, additives, or new oak" comes from a larger vision of building a legacy for his family. More than a decade ago, the family home that sat on what is now the vineyard burned down, taking with it a generation of family heirlooms and memories. James decided to create something new for the family, an organic farm and vineyard to honor his father, Frank. The first certified organic winery in Idaho, Holesinsky turned heads when the 22-year-old James planted his first Chardonnay grapes in 2000. Now he is working with biodynamic practices as well, and the vineyard has grown to 12 acres, with an additional 4 acres at another site. Plantings include Syrah, Merlot, Cabernet Sauvignon, Riesling, and Muscat, as well as Souzão, Tinta Cão, and Touriga Nacional grapes for his port-style wine. With his University of California at Davis Extension training, mentoring from some of Washington State's best, such as Rick Small of Woodward Canyon, and his commitment to a family dream, Holesinsky is well on his way to creating a legacy for Idaho wine.

Wines to Try: The Original Riesling is made in a slightly off-dry style, with white blossom and apple notes, and bright acidity that makes it refreshing with salads, fish, and poultry, and dynamite with fruit.

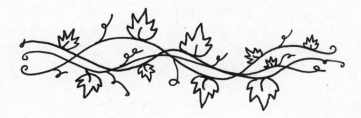

OTHER IDAHO WINERIES WITH GREEN CONSIDERATIONS

COEUR D'ALENE CELLARS
3890 N. Schreiber Way
Coeur d'Alene, ID 83815
(208) 664-2336
www.cdacellars.com
SS (Stillwater Creek Syrah)

KOENIG DISTILLERY AND WINERY
20928 Grape Lane
Caldwell, ID 83607
(208) 455-8386
www.koenigdistilleryandwinery
.com

SAWTOOTH WINERY
13750 Surrey Lane
Nampa, ID 83686
(208) 467-1200
www.sawtoothwinery.com

BRITISH COLUMBIA WINERIES

British Columbia's winemakers and growers are very intercon-nected, probably because the community is relatively small, with winegrowers working for various vineyards and sharing knowledge. The biggest wine region is the Okanagan, with about 65 wineries (about 15 certified organic or transitioning) and approximately 143 organic acres planted. The area, about two hours north of central Washington State, is a gorgeous place to take a wine vacation. It is situated on the banks of Lake Okanagan, which helps regulate vine-yard temperatures and mitigate freezes. A hidden gem of a region, it produces excellent wines, which range from cool-climate Pinot Gris, Gewürztraminer, and Pinot Noir along the Naramata Bench near Kelowna, to Cabernet Sauvignon, Merlot, and even Syrah in the southern Osoyoos area. Organic standards are set by the Certified

Organic Associations of British Columbia (COABC), and sustainable farming has been adopted faster here than in many areas of the North American wine industry.

BURROWING OWL WINERY
100 Burrowing Owl Place · Oliver, BC, V0H 1T0, Canada
(250) 498-0620 · www.burrowingowl.com

At Burrowing Owl, named after one of the true icons of the BC wine region, proceeds from the tasting room go to benefit owl conservation. Jim Wyse planted his vineyard in 1993 on the Black Sage Bench, creating only the highest-quality Cabernet Sauvignon, Cabernet Franc, Merlot, Chardonnay, and even Pinot Gris and Pinot Noir from his estate vineyard. Situated at the tip of the Sonora Desert, this 140-acre vineyard is a "deceptively fragile desert ecosystem, and is a continual challenge" for the Burrowing Owls team. They have taken many steps to avoid using pesticides and herbicides, such as installing 100-plus bluebird boxes and two bat nurseries to encourage those animals to help with pest populations. They also power their tasting room, restaurant, swimming pool, and inn with solar and geothermal electricity. The beautiful inn with great food makes a great place to start a wine tour of the Okanagan.

DEEP CREEK WINE ESTATE/HAINLE VINEYARDS ESTATE WINERY CO
5355 Trepanier Bench Road · Peachland, BC, V0H 1X2, Canada
(250) 212-5944 · www.hainle.com

The 18-acre Hainle Estate Vineyards on the shore of Lake Okanagan has been certified organic since 1992. This winery has the distinction of being the first winery to create an organic ice wine in North America, when owner Walter Hainle, in a nod to his German heritage, used frozen grapes to make wine rather than waste them, releasing his first ice wine in 1978. Now, winemaker Jason Parkes continues to make ice wine and other award-winning wines. According to the operation's organic information, in 1995 it brought Traminer, Riesling, Bibendum white, Bibendum rosé, and ice wine into certified organic production for the first time in BC. Organic vineyards often have lower yields, which is one reason this method appeals to winemakers, but, according to Parkes, "labor costs, particularly for soil improvement and weed control, are higher. Some growers have found that the reduced yields mean better plant health and better fruit quality, bringing higher per-ton returns that help to offset the increased labor costs. For other growers, this equation may not work. Each grower makes his or her own decision. Each vineyard and each grower has a distinct personality."

JOIE FARM
Not certified, organic practices
Naramata, British Columbia
(866) 422-5643 · www.joiefarm.com
No tasting room

Heidi Noble and Michael Dinn have a small, 5-acre vineyard on the Naramata Bench that grows Gewürztraminer and Yellow Muscat, but they work with other vineyards to grow grapes for their delicious wines. They plant cover crops as nitrogen fixers, including mustards, vetch, white and red clover, and wildflowers. They use an extremely small amount of water, watering once in the spring and then again only in extreme heat situations, in order to let the vines strengthen their root systems. "[V]iticulture is not a textbook practice, but a process of constant observation," says Michael, and the pair walks their vineyard daily, so that they can spot and be on top of any problems that might occur.

Wines to Try: Joie Farm wines are elegant, fresh, and well balanced and are mostly sold through a private mailing list and Vancouver and

Victoria area restaurants (look for them there, if you get a chance). One favorite is A Noble Blend, which usually includes several traditional Alsatian grapes such as Riesling, Gewürztraminer, Pinot Blanc, Pinot Auxerrois, and Schönberger, and is a bit off-dry with all sorts of floral and spice aromas, and tropical fruits such as lychee and guava, with a zesty lime peel finish.

ROLLINGDALE WINERY
CO
2306 Hayman Road · West Kelowna, BC, V1Z 1Z5, Canada
(250) 769-9224 · www.rollingdalewinery.com

Awarded Best Organic Winery of 2010 by *Organic Wine Review*, this Kelowna winery is owned by Steve and Kristy Dale, who make a premium estate-grown, certified organic Pinot Gris ice wine and also a Pinot Noir ice wine, which is quite unusual. Winemaker Joe Slykerman and vineyard manager Kyp Rowe focus on the highest quality grapes they can get: "It is important we let consumers know that our wine is not loaded with impurities," says owner Steve Dale. They source a lot of fruit from Okanagan vineyards, and some barrels from Okanagan Barrel Works; these barrels, assembled from French oak in BC, save thousands of miles' worth of fuel and emissions over shipping barrels from France.

SUMMERHILL PYRAMID WINERY
CO
4870 Chute Lake Road · Kelowna, BC, V1W 4M3, Canada
(250) 764-8000 · www.summerhill.bc.ca

Stephen and Wendy Cipes and partner Eric von Krosigk started Summerhill in 1991 and have been passionate leaders in educating wine lovers about organic wine ever since. They are very transparent about their process and have great educational tools on their website comparing conventional winegrowing and winemaking to organic and to their own processes, including which additives they use in the wines and why. Their minimal manipulation process is top priority, and with the semidesert climate, the vineyards flourish. Vineyard manager Harold Gaudy is a "dry-farming, pesticide-hating, French-speaking, ground-cover-loving, leaf-plucking, convention-shunning vine whisperer," and the team, which also includes Cipes sons Ezra and Gabe, along with chef Jesse Croy, has created an organic farm-to-glass winery that celebrates the purity of the fruit they grow. A tour of Summerhill includes tasting the award-winning organically grown wines, lunch or dinner in the Sunset Organic Bistro, and a visit to the Summerhill Pyramid, which was built as a place to enjoy peace and tranquility. Stephen says, "I recently started a little experiment, asking the tours to turn off their cell phones and to take a few moments of their busy lives to just *be*." To the Cipeses, this land, with its roots in Westbank First Nation heritage, is a sacred historical place. The site features a settler's cabin and the Makwala Kekuli, a replica of a First Nation winter house that you can tour.

TINHORN CREEK   LIVE · SS
32830 Tinhorn Creek Road · Oliver, BC, V0H 1T0, Canada
(250) 498-3743 · (888) 484-6467 · www.tinhorn.com

Started by friends Kenn Oldfield and Bob Shaunessey with barrels of wine in a basement, Tinhorn Creek now encompasses 150 acres of grapes on two sites, the cooler Tinhorn Creek Vineyard, near the winery in South Okanagan's Golden Mile region, and the Diamondback Vineyard, on the hotter Black Sage Bench. Vineyard manager Andrew Moon uses common sense in the vineyard, composting pomace and moving to drip irrigation rather than spraying water. Instead of spraying or baiting pests, he eliminates large rocks and other hiding places, utilizes snake fences, and encourages beneficial predators with habitat such as bluebird boxes. Ninety percent of the glass (about half of which is recycled) is made within about 300 miles of the winery. The site also includes a concert venue and a restaurant, Miradoro, that makes a trip to Tinhorn Creek especially enjoyable.

Wines to Try: Winemaker Sandra Oldfield says she has only about "40 or 50 opportunities [in her life] to make the best Merlot—overall, that's really not that many." That made me curious to try these wines, knowing that the dry, sunny climate of the Okanagan makes it a great region for this lush grape, helping retain its acidity and balance. Oldfield adds a bit of Cabernet Franc and Syrah to highlight the earthiness of this unique Merlot.

OTHER BRITISH COLUMBIA WINERIES WITH GREEN CONSIDERATIONS

FORBIDDEN FRUIT WINERY
620 Sumac Road
Cawston, BC, V0X 1C3, Canada
(250) 499-2649
www.forbiddenfuitwines.com
Art gallery
CO

LA STELLA WINERY
8123 148th Avenue, RR 2
Osoyoos, BC, V0H 1V2, Canada
(250) 495-8180
www.lastella.ca
Low-input viticulture

LE VIEUX PIN
5496 Black Sage Road
Oliver, BC, V0H 1T0, Canada
(250) 498-8388
www.levieuxpin.ca
Low-input viticulture

RUSTIC ROOTS
2238 Highway 3
Cawston, BC, V0X 1C2, Canada
(250) 499.2754
www.rusticrootswinery.com
Fruit wines
CO

Green Vine Resources

BOOKS

Chartier, François. *Taste Buds and Molecules: The Art and Science of Food, Wine and Flavor*. Hoboken, NJ: John Wiley & Sons, Inc., 2012.

Chauvet, Jules. *Le Vin en Question*. Paris: Jean-Paul Rocher, 1998.

Cole, Katherine. *Voodoo Vintners: Oregon's Astonishing Biodynamic Winegrowers*. Corvallis, OR: Oregon State University Press, 2011.

Feiring, Alice. *Naked Wine: Letting Grapes Do What Comes Naturally*. Cambridge, MA: Da Capo Press, 2011.

Goode, Jamie, and Sam Harrop. *Authentic Wine: Toward Natural and Sustainable Winemaking*. Berkeley, CA: University of California Press, 2011.

Grahm, Randall. *Been Doon So Long: A Randall Grahm Vinthology*. Berkeley, CA: University of California Press, 2012.

Joly, Nicolas. *Biodynamic Wine, Demystified*. San Francisco: Wine Appreciation Guild, 2008.

———. *What Is Biodynamic Wine? The Quality, the Taste, the Terroir*. East Sussex, UK: Clairview Books, 2012.

———. *Wine from Sky to Earth: Growing & Appreciating Biodynamic Wine*. Austin, TX: Acres USA, 2005.

Katz, Sandor Ellix, and Michael Pollan. *The Art of Fermentation: An In-Depth Exploration of Essential Concepts and Processes from Around the World*. White River Junction, VT: Chelsea Green, 2012.

Matthews, Patrick. *Real Wine: The Rediscovery of Natural Winemaking*. London: Mitchell Beazley, 2000.

Scully, Matthew. *Dominion: The Power of Man, the Suffering of Animals, and the Call to Mercy*. New York: St. Martin's Press, 2002.

Waldin, Monty. *Biodynamic Wines*. London: Mitchell Beazley, 2004.

ONLINE RESOURCES AND WEBSITES FOR FURTHER READING

Biodynamic Farming and Gardening Association
www.biodynamics.com
A great resource for information about biodynamics. They publish *The Biodynamic Directory*, an online members-only resource for biodynamic products and resources.

Center for Columbia River History

www.ccrh.org

An interesting source for the history of Washington State agriculture and water issues.

Eric Texier Wines

www.donkeyandagoat.com/texier/home.htm

Information about French natural winemaker Eric Texier and his wines.

The Feiring Line

www.alicefeiring.com

A captivating blog by New York writer Alice Feiring that explores issues surrounding the natural wine movement, among other fascinating aspects of wine.

French natural wine

www.morethanorganic.com

The website of Pierre Jancou, a French "cook, restaurant owner, wine merchant, and importer of natural wines" living in Paris.

Holdren, John P., Gretchen C. Daily, and Paul R. Ehrlich. *The Meaning of Sustainability: Biogeophysical Aspects*. Washington, DC: The United Nations University, 1995. dieoff.org/page113.htm.

Natural wines information

www.foodtourist.com

Links to articles on the natural wine movement.

Roza Irrigation District

www.roza.org

Information about the history of the Yakima River irrigation project.

Rudolph Steiner College

www.steinercollege.edu

A college in Fair Oaks, California, teaching Waldorf Teacher Education, biodynamics, and the philosophy of Rudolph Steiner.

Thrupp, L. Ann, Michael J. Costello, and Glenn McGourty. *Biodiversity Conservation Practices in California Vineyards: Learning from Experiences*. San Francisco: California Sustainable Winegrowing Program, 2008. www.sustainablewinegrowing.org/docs/2008-Biodiversity_in_Vineyards.pdf.

US Department of Agriculture. *Guidelines for Labeling: Wine with Organic References*. Washington, DC: USDA, 2009. www.ttb.gov/pdf/wine.pdf.

CERTIFYING AGENCIES, REGIONAL WINE COMMISSIONS, AND GROWER ORGANIZATIONS

British Columbia Wine Institute
www.winebc.org
The Wine Institute is a consumer organization that promotes wines from British Columbia.

British Columbia Grapegrowers Association
www.grapegrowers.bc.ca
British Columbia's education and promotional organization for grape growers.

California Association of Winegrape Growers
www.cawg.org
Promotes environmentally friendly practices in the California wine industry.

California Certified Organic Farmers
www.ccof.org
Promotes and supports organic agriculture in California and elsewhere through an organic certification program, education, and advocacy.

California Sustainable Winegrowing Alliance
www.sustainablewinegrowing.org
Supports California growers and the California Sustainable Winegrowing Program certification.

Central Coast Vineyard Team
www.vineyardteam.org
A nonprofit grower group that promotes sustainable vineyard practices in Santa Barbara, San Luis Obispo, Monterey, Santa Cruz, and San Benito counties.

Deep Roots Coalition
www.facebook.com/pages/Deep-Roots-Coalition/125656974183606
A small group of Oregon winegrowers who promote the practice of dry farming and educate consumers about the benefits and authenticity of wine produced without irrigation.

Delinat Institute
www.delinat-institut.org
A revolutionary Swiss organization that studies "climate positive" farming with high biodiversity at its vineyard in Valais, Switzerland.

Demeter International
www.demeter.net
www.demeter-usa.org
Demeter International is HQ for all things biodynamic. Demeter-USA is the center for biodynamic certification and education in the United States. Demeter also

has an organic certification process, Stellar Certification, so farms that are Demeter Certified Biodynamic can become USDA Certified Organic at the same time.

Fish Friendly Farming
www.fishfriendlyfarming.org
A voluntary certification program for California grape growers who implement land management practices that restore and sustain fish habitat.

The Food Alliance
foodalliance.org
A nonprofit organization that promotes sustainable agriculture and educates consumers about its benefits.

Idaho Wine Commission
www.idahowines.org
Idaho's consumer education organization promoting the Idaho wine industry.

The Lodi Rules for Sustainable Winegrowing
www.lodiwine.com/certified-green
California's first third-party certification program for winegrowing.

Low Input Viticulture and Enology (LIVE)
www.liveinc.org
A program that certifies vineyards and wineries for sustainable agricultural practices modeled after international standards.

Napa Sustainable Winegrowing Group
www.naparcd.org/nswg.html
An organization whose mission is to identify and promote winegrowing practices that are economically viable, socially responsible, and environmentally sound.

Oregon Certified Sustainable Wine
www.ocsw.org
A consumer education organization that promotes wineries with the LIVE and Salmon-Safe Certifications.

Oregon Tilth Certified Organic
tilth.org
A nonprofit research and education organization dedicated to biologically sound and socially equitable agriculture.

Oregon Wine Board
www.oregonwine.org
Oregon's consumer resource for information about the state's wine industry.

Oregon Winegrowers Association
www.oregonwinegrowers.org
Supports Oregon growers through education and advocacy.

Renaissance des Appellations (Return to Terroir)
www.return-to-terroir.com
An international organic/biodynamic organization whose members adhere to strict organic and quality standards, based in Savennières, France.

Salmon-Safe
www.salmonsafe.org
Certification program in the Pacific Northwest providing recognition for agricultural operations that work to conserve resources and maintain viable runs of salmon and steelhead.

Sonoma County Winegrape Commission
www.sonomawinegrape.org
Provides resources and support for growers in Sonoma and Marin counties, California.

Stewardship Partners
www.stewardshippartners.org
A conservation group that promotes the Salmon-Safe certification and works to restore the watersheds of Washington State and Puget Sound.

USDA National Organic Program
www.ams.usda.gov/AMSv1.0/nop
The US Department of Agriculture's website for information on the organic certification program.

Vinea: The Winegrowers' Sustainable Trust
www.vineatrust.com
Washington's sustainable winegrowing organization, using LIVE standards for certification.

Vinewise: The Washington Guide to Sustainable Viticulture
www.vinewise.org
The Vinewise Guide is a series of self-evaluation forms for grape growers covering specific sustainable viticulture and business topics.

Washington Association of Wine Grape Growers
www.wawgg.org
Supports the Washington winegrowing industry through education and promotion.

Washington Wine Commission

www.washingtonwine.org

Washington's consumer education organization promoting the state's wine industry.

Wine Institute

www.wineinstitute.org

Promotes the California wine industry and co-sponsors the California Sustainable Winegrowing Program along with the California Association of Winegrape Growers.

Winerywise: The Washington Guide to Sustainable Winery Practices

www.winerywise.org

Winerywise is a self-assessment program for winemakers to evaluate and improve their sustainable practices throughout the winemaking process.

CONSUMER INFORMATION

American Tartaric Products

www.americantartaric.com

Sells processing aids and additives for wine.

Community Alliance with Family Farmers

www.caff.org

A California nonprofit member-activist organization fostering family-scale agriculture that cares for the land, sustains local economies, and promotes social justice.

Consumers Union Guide to Environmental Labels

www.eco-labels.org

A source for information about labels and certifications for consumers.

FoodHub

www.food-hub.org

A project of EcoTrust: a searchable database of farmers, ranchers, fishermen, and food manufacturers in the Pacific Northwest.

Organic Consumers Association

www.organicconsumers.org

A clearinghouse for information on organic products.

SUSTAINABLE PRACTICES FOR WINE AND BEYOND

Cascades Raptor Center

www.eraptors.org

This organization based in Eugene, Oregon, rescues and releases raptors, including some in agricultural areas to help reduce rodent populations.

Cork Forest Conservation Alliance

www.corkforest.org

A leader in the cork recycling movement and campaigner for the preservation of cork forests (formerly Cork ReHarvest).

Eco-Glass

www.eco-glass.org

A company that produces lighter wine bottles from recycled glass.

The Hungry Owl Project

www.hungryowl.org

A nonprofit based in Marin County, California, that releases owls into agricultural areas to help reduce the need for rodenticides and pesticides.

Leadership in Energy and Environmental Design (LEED)

new.usgbc.org

A certification program for architecture through the US Green Building Council.

ReCORK

recork.org

An international cork recycling program for natural wine corks.

Salud!

www.saludauction.org

A healthcare organization for Oregon's seasonal vineyard workers and their families, supported by an annual auction put on by Oregon wineries.

SOLE

www.yoursole.com

A shoe company that uses recycled cork in some of its products.

Tetra Pak

www.tetrapak.com

Producers of collapsible packaging for wine and other consumables.

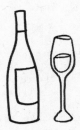

Index

3 Horse Ranch Vineyards, 187

A to Z Wineworks, 117
Abacela, 118
Abeja, 37, 153
additives, 41
Adelsheim Vineyard, 119
àMaurice Cellars, 38, 154
Amavi Cellars, 155
Ambyth Estate, 91
Amity Vineyards, 120
Ampelos Cellars, 112
Anam Cara Cellars, 120
Anderson, Joy, 167, 174
Angel Vine Wine, 150
Anne Amie Vineyards, 121
Antica Terra, 147
Araujo Estate Wines, 92
ArborBrook Vineyards, 147
Arbor Crest Wine Cellars, 182
Argyle Winery, 121

Badger Mountain Vineyard, 156
Baer Winery, 182
Bainbridge Island Vineyards & Winery,
    158
Baron, Christophe, 159
Barra of Mendocino, 92
Baumé, 27
Beaver Creek Vineyards, 93
Beaux Frères, 147
Beckmen Vineyards, 112
Beckmeyer, Hank, 19, 106
Bee Friendly Farming (BFF), 80
Belle Pente, 147
Benton-Lane Vineyard, 122
bentonite, 41
Benziger Family Winery, 94, 109
Beresan Winery, 182
Bethel Heights Vineyard, 123
Bergström Wines, 124

Beveridge, Paul, 33, 179, 181
biodynamics
    definition, 32, 59
    preparations, 33, 59–60, 181
Bishop Creek Cellars, 125
Bitner Winery, 183, 187
Bjornstad Cellars, 112
Black Sears Estate Wines, 112
Bonny Doon Vineyard, 21, 94, 172
Bonterra Organic Vineyards, 95
Bookwalter, 183
Bourguignon, Claude, 34
Boushey, Dick, 177–178
Brick House Vineyards, 70, 125
Brittan Vineyards, 148
Brooks, 145, 148
Brooks, Jimi, 144
Bucklin, 96
Burrowing Owl Winery, 191
Buty Winery, 37, 159
Bybee Vineyards & Habitat, 113

Cain, Matthew, 50
California Certified Organic Farmers
    (CCOF), 30, 65, 198
California Sustainable Winegrowing
    Alliance (CCSW), 68–70,
Cameron Winery, 126
Canadian Food Inspection Agency
    (CFIA), 61
Carbon Neutral Challenge, 46, 71, 141
Cardwell Hill Cellars, 148
Carlton Cellars, 148
Cascade Raptor Center, 146
casein, 41
Casteel, Ted, 123
Cayuse Vineyards, 153, 157, 159
Ceago Vinegarden, 97
Ceritas Wines, 113
Chartier, François, 78–79
Chateau Ste. Michelle, 160, 167

Chauncey, Joe, 178–179
Chauvet, Jules, 43
Chehalem, 127
Chelan Estate Winery, 183
China Bend Winery, 161
Chinook Winery, 183
Cinder Wines, 188
Claar Cellars, 162
Cline, Phil, 179, 181
Clubb, Marty, 167
Coehlo Winery, 148
Coeur D'Alene Cellars, 190
Cole, Katherine, 34
Concha y Toro, 102
conventional farming, 28–29
Constellation Brands, 47
Cooper Mountain Winery, 128
cork, 49, 81, 146, 180, 202
Cork Forest Conservation Alliance, 49, 202
Côte Bonneville, 183
Coturri Winery, 113
Covington Cellars, 183
Cowhorn, 128
Cristom, 129
Custer, Danielle, 77

Davero, 98
Deep Creek Wine Estate, 191
Deep Roots Coalition, 21, 38
de Lancellotti Family Vineyards, 124
DeLoach Vineyards, 99
Demeter Certified Biodynamic, 33, 42, 45, 58, 59
Demeter (USA & International), 56, 140, 198
Dobbes Family Estate, 130
Dobbes, Joe, 130
Domaine Danielle Laurent, 129
Domaine de la Romanée-Conti, 39
Domaine Drouhin, 130
Domaine Serene, 132
Dominio IV, 148
Donkey & Goat, 113

Drouhin, Véronique, 130
dry farming, 21
Dumol, 113
Dunham Cellars, 162

Eco-Glass, 49
Ehlers Estate, 101
Elizabeth Spencer Wines, 115
Elk Cove Vineyards, 132
Eola Hills, 148
Erath, Dick, 116
Evening Land Vineyards, 133
Evesham Wood, 134
Eyrie Vineyards, 148

Fetzer, 101–102
Fetzer, Jim, 97
Feiring, Alice, 42
Figgins Family Wine Estate, 163
fine, 41
Fish Friendly Farming (FFF), 70
Five Star Cellars, 183
flavor management, 43
Food Alliance (FA), 72
Forbidden Fruit Winery, 195
Four Graces, 148
Freemark Abbey, 103
Frey Vineyards, 30, 98, 103
Frog's Leap Winery, 104
Fukuoka, Masanobu, 107

Garrison Creek Cellars Estate Vineyard and Winery, 183
Gilbert Cellars, 164
Glacial Lake Missoula, 19
Gorman Winery, 183
Grahm, Randall, 21, 88, 172
gravity flow, 47
greenwashing, 66–67
Grgich Hills Estate, 105
Grgich, Mike, 105
Gross, Robert and Corrine, 128
Guardian Cellars, 184

Haber process, 29
Haden Fig, 134
Hainle Vineyards Estate Winery, 191
Hall Winery, 47
Hawk and Horse Vineyards, 106
Hedges, Christophe, 157, 164
Hedges Family Estate Winery, 157, 164
Heibel Ranch Vineyards, 113
Hightower Cellars, 165
Hobo Wine Company, 113
Holesinsky Certified Organic Vineyard
    and Winery, 189
Hollywood Hill Vineyards, 166
Hungry Owl Project, 202

Illahe Vineyards, 148
inputs, 29, 42
International Organization for Biological
    and Integrated Control (IOBC), 55, 57
Isinglass, 41

JM Cellars, 184
Januik Winery, 171
Jeriko Estate, 113
Johan Vineyards, 134
Joie Farm, 192
Joly, Nicolas, 35, 181
Jordan Vineyards & Winery, 113

Kamen Estate Wines, 113
King Estate Winery, 135
Klipsun Vineyard, 69
Koenig Distillery and Winery, 190
Kramer, Matt, 17, 25, 70
Kramer Vineyards, 149

La Clarine Farm, 19, 106
Lange Estate Winery, 149
La Stella Winery, 195
Latah Creek, 184
Leaders in Energy and Environmental
    Design (LEED), 45, 47, 81, 143, 178
L'Ecole No. 41, 167
Left Coast Cellars, 136

Lemelson Vineyards, 136
Leonetti Cellar, 163
Lett, David, 116
Le Vieux Pin, 195
Littorai Wines, 107
locavore, 135
Lodi Rules for Sustainable Winegrowing
    Certified Green (LR), 81
Long Meadow Ranch Winery, 114
Lopez Island Winery, 169
Low Input Viticulture and Enology
    (LIVE), 73
Lullaby Winery, 184
Lumos Wine Company, 138
Lutea Wine Cellars, 114

Maboroshi Wine Estates, 114
Mahonia Vineyards, 138
malolactic fermentation, 44
Mark Ryan Winery, 184
Masquerade Cellars, 184
Masút Vineyard and Winery, 114
Matthews Cellars, 184
Maysara Winery, 139
McKibben, Norm, 75, 173
Memaloose, 169
Mendocino Valley, 98
Mendocino Wine Company, 100, 108
Merry Cellars, 184
minerality, 12, 26–27, 88
Molecular Sommellerie, 77–80
Momtazi Vineyard, 139
Montemaggiore, 114
Montinore Estate, 140

Naches Heights Vineyard, 170
Napa Green (NG), 71
Narrow Gate Vineyards, 114
natural wine, 41
noninterventionist philosophy, 107
Nora's Table, 137
Northstar Winery, 184
Nota Bene Cellars, 185
Novelty Hill Winery, 36, 37, 171

Oregon Certified Sustainable Wine (OCSW), 74
Oregon Tilth Certified Organic (OTCO), 64, 65, 199
organic, definition, 62
Owen Roe, 149

Pacific Rim, 172
Panther Creek Cellars, 149
Parducci Wine Cellars, 108
Parkerization, 157
Patianna Organic Vineyards, 114
Patton Valley Vineyard, 149
Paul Dolan Vineyards, 100
Paul, John, 39, 126
Pellet, Jean-François, 171
Penner-Ash Wine Cellars, 149
Pepper Bridge, 37, 167, 173
pest management, 33
Pogue, Kevin, 20
Ponzi Vineyards, 149
Porter-Bass Winery, 114
Porter Creek Vineyards, 114
Portteus, 185
Powers, Bill, 30
Powers Winery, 152, 156
Preston Vineyards, 115
proprietary vineyard programs, 122, 132
Puma Springs Vineyards, 109

Quintessa, 115
Quivira Vineyards & Winery, 110

Radio-Coteau, 115
Rainforest Alliance Forest Stewardship Council (FSC), 81
Raymond Vineyards, 115
ReCORK, 49, 180
Redford, Myron, 120
Reininger Winery, 185
Rex Hill Vineyards, 117, 149
Robert Sinskey Vineyards, 111
Rolland, Michel, 92

Rollingdale Winery, 193
Rustic Roots, 195

Salmon-Safe (SS), 35, 75
Salud!, 142
Saviah Cellars, 185
Sawtooth Winery, 190
Schafer, Anna, 37
Score Revolution Manifesto, 157
Seguin, Gérard, 27
Seven Hills Winery, 185
Shafer Vineyards, 110
Sineann, 149
Slow Food, 43
Small, Rick, 180
Snoqualmie Vineyards, 165, 174
Sokol Blosser, 140
solar energy, 47
SOLE, 51
Soles, Rollin, 121
Sommer, Richard, 116
Sonoma County Winegrape Commission (SCWC), 82
Soter Vineyards, 141
Spindrift Cellars, 149
spinning cone, 43
Spoiled Dog Winery, 175
Steiner, Rudolph, 32, 35, 59, 107, 181, 197
Stewardship Partners, 36, 75, 200
Stillwater Creek Vineyard, 36
Stoller Vineyards, 127, 143
sulfite free, 63, 128
Summerhill Pyramid Winery, 193
sustainability, 22
Syncline, 185

Tagaris Winery, 185
Tamarack Cellars, 185
Tempus Cellars, 185
Terra Blanca Winery & Estate Vineyard, 176
Territorial Vineyards & Wine Company, 150

Tertulia Cellars, 185
TetraPak, 49, 99
Texier, Eric, 43
Three Angels Vineyard, 150
Tinhorn Creek, 194
Topel Winery, 115
Torii Mor Winery, 150
Trillium Creek Winery, 186
Trium Winery, 150
Troon Vineyard, 150
Truett Hurst, 115
Tunnell, Doug, 67, 125–126, 129
Two Mountain Winery, 176
Tyee Wine Cellars, 150

Unti Vineyards, 115
Upchurch, Chris, 177
Upchurch Vineyard, 177
Urban Wine Works, 125
USDA Certified Organic, 62–64

Van Duzer Vineyards, 144
Va Piano Vineyards, 31, 186
Verge, 115
verjus, 85
Viader, 116
Vidon Vineyard, 145
Vinea, 76
VineWise, 152
Vino-Lok, 50
vin naturel, 44
vins d'effort, 11

vins de terroir, 11
Vista Hills Vineyard & Winery, 150
VML Winery, 116

Wallula Vineyard, 89, 172
Watermill Winery, 150
Waters, 178
Westport Winery, 186
Westrey Wine Company, 151
Wild Hog Vineyard, 116
Wild Salmon Center, 172
WillaKenzie Estate, 142, 151
Willamette Valley Vineyards, 146
Wilridge Winery, 179, 181
Winderlea Vineyard & Winery, 147
winemaking process, 40
Winerywise, 153, 167
Winter's Hill Vineyard, 151
Witness Tree Vineyard, 151
Woodinville Wine Cellars, 186
Woodward Canyon, 180
Wooldridge Creek Vineyard & Winery,
  151

Yakima Project, 23
Yellow+Blue, 50
York, Alan, 94, 129
Yorkville Cellars, 116
Youngberg Hill, 151

Zerba Cellars, 151

About the Author

Shannon Borg is a writer, wine educator, poet, and editor. She has written about food, wine, spirits, and beer for magazines and websites including *Seattle* magazine,

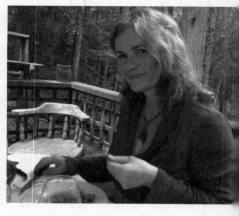

Northwest Palate, Wine Press Northwest, Northwest Brewing News, AvalonWine.com, and CitySearch.com. She co-authored a cookbook, *Chefs on the Farm: Recipes and Inspiration from the Quillisascut Farm School of the Domestic Arts* (Skipstone, 2008). Certified by the International Sommelier Guild (Wine Fundamentals I & II), Shannon is the sommelier for Doe Bay Café at Doe Bay Resort and Retreat on Orcas Island in Washington State.

In addition to her extensive food and wine credentials, Shannon holds an MFA in poetry from the University of Washington and a PhD in poetry and literature from the University of Houston. She has taught writing at the University of Houston, Seattle Art Institute, Richard Hugo House, and Spokane Community College. Her poems have been published in numerous journals including the *Paris Review, London Review of Books, Poetry Northwest, Gulf Coast, Cranky, Indiana Review,* and *Antioch Review.* Her book of poems, *Corset,* was published by Cherry Grove in 2006.

Follow Shannon on her blog, www.shannonborg.wordpress.com, as she hatches new writing projects.